INTUITIVE EATING

Think Intuitively! Developing a healthy relationship towards food.

Stop unnecessary craving and say YES to INTUITIVE EATING

By Manuel Nestor Eagle

Copyright © 2019 Manuel Nestor Eagle

All rights reserved. No part of this publication may be reproduced, distributed, or transmitted in any form or by any means, including photocopying, recording, or other electronic or mechanical methods, without the prior written permission of the publisher, except in the case of brief quotations embodied in critical reviews and certain other noncommercial uses permitted by copyright law.

Table Of Contents

Introduction 1

Chapter 1: Understanding the concept of intuitive eating 6

Chapter 2: Dieter's headache 13

Chapter 3: Thinking like an intuitive eater 28

Chapter 4: Know the kind of eater you are 42

Chapter 5: Separating emotions & hunger 49

Chapter 6: The First Principle: Reject the Diet Mentality 65

Chapter 7: The Second principle: Honor your Hunger 75

Chapter 8: The Third Principle – Be Content with Nourishment 84

Chapter 9: The Fourth Principle – Challenging the Food Police. 94

Chapter 10: The Fifth Principles: Respect Your Fullness 103

Chapter 11: The Sixth Principle: Discover the Satisfaction Factor 113

Chapter 12: The Seventh Principle: Honor Your Feeling Without Using Food 124

Chapter 13: The Eighth Principle: Respect Your Body. 133

Chapter 14: The Ninth Principle: Exercise- Feel the Difference 142

Chapter 15: The Tenth Principle: Honor Your Health with Gentle Nutrition 148

Chapter 16: Confusion About Nutrition 153

Chapter 17: Scientists Thoughts on Intuitive Eating 176

Chapter 18: Putting Intuitive Diet into Practice 191

Conclusion 201

Introduction

Intuitive eating is the ideal thought of eating what makes you the master of your body and its craving signals.

Basically, it's something contrary to a conventional eating regimen. It doesn't force rules about maintaining a strategic distance from and when or what to eat.

Rather, it gives you that mentality that you are the best individual — the only individual — to settle on those decisions.

Intuitive eating is an eating style that builds a sound frame of mind toward nourishment and self-perception.

The thought is that you ought to eat when you're hungry and stop when you're full.

Even though this should be an intuitive procedure, for some individuals, it's most certainly not.

Believing diet books so-called specialists about what, when, and how to nourish your body can lead you from confiding in your body and its instinct.

To eat naturally, you may need to relearn how to confide in your body. To do that, you have to recognize physical and emotional appetite:

- **Physical hunger:** This organic urge instructs you to recharge supplements. It promotes step by step and has various sign, for example, fatigue, a growling stomach, or irritability. It's fulfilled when you eat any nourishment.
- **Emotional hunger:** This is driven by enthusiastic need. Misery, dejection, and boredom are a portion of the emotions that can make yearnings for food, frequently comfort nourishments. Eating at that point causes self-loathing and guilt.

Intuitive eating is tied in with believing your internal body wisdom to settle on decisions around nourishment that generate great vibe in your body, without judgment and impact from diet culture. We are altogether brought into the world with the aptitude to eat, to stop when we are full, to eat when we are ravenous, and to eat fulfilling nourishments. As we grow up, that can change for various reasons. A large number of us lose that opportunity, and intuitive eating is figuring out how to recover it. At the point when we channel out the clamour and impact that diet culture presents to us as false facts, we can then really tune in to what our body needs and wants from nourishment.

Intuitive eating is a harmonious development. It's about stopping the war with your body, figuring out how to acknowledge our different hereditary outlines. Diet culture would have us accept every one of the guidelines we have around nourishment as gospel since they are all, here and there, concentrated on the dainty perfect; that anyone other than a slight one, isn't right. Those nourishment rules lead to an enthusiastic worth put on nourishment, and when we put that passionate incentive on nourishment, we at that point disguise it as we eat, and that prompts thoughts like, "I'm so terrible due to the fact that I ate XXXXXX."

Let me get straight to the point; food/nourishment isn't positive or negative, and naming it in that capacity can present numerous issues. Healthfully, much the same as bodies, all nourishments are extraordinary. Genuinely, all nourishments must be equivalent. One nourishment doesn't make you terrible, while a different one makes you great. In the event that we can approach ALL FOODS as genuinely comparable, we can really start to associate with our very own inward astuteness. Intuitive eating is tied in with causing harmony with nourishment and surrendering the unnecessary war against our body and the way we eat.

Intuitive eating is testing and can hard to get it. It's the direct inverse of how we've been instructed to consider nourishment. It's not dark or white, it's dim, nuanced and there is nobody's "right way" which is the reason it tends to be so confounding.

Intuitive eating is a beautiful piece of recuperation. It is likewise a fundamental piece in the aversion of dietary problems. In the event that you are battling to comprehend what intuitive eating truly is.

Chapter 1: Understanding the concept of intuitive eating

Intuitive eating is a methodology that was made by two enrolled dietitians, Evelyn Tribole and Elyse Resch, in 1995. Intuitive eating is a non-diet way to deal with wellbeing and health that causes you to tune into your body signals, break the cycle of interminable eating fewer carbs, and mend your association with nourishment. From a proficient diet viewpoint, intuitive eating is a structure that encourages us to keep food mediations conduct centred rather than restricting or rule-centred.

We are altogether brought into the world regular natural eaters. Children cry, they eat, and afterward quit eating until they're ravenous once more. Children inherently equal out their nourishment admission from week to week, eating when they're hungry and halting once they feel full. A few days, they may eat a massive amount of nourishment, and different days they may eat anything scarcely. As we become more established and rules and confinements are set around food, we lose our inward instinctive eater. We figure out how to finish everything on our plate. We discover that treat is a reward or can be removed in the event that we act mischievously. We are informed that specific nourishments are beneficial for us, and others are terrible – making us like ourselves when we eat certain nourishments and feeling terrible when we eat others.

Intuitive eating isn't an eating routine. Actually, it's the inverse. There's no checking calories or macros and no creation of certain limits for food. It's not tied in with moving along with a meal plan or allotting your portions (truth be told, that is altogether disheartened!). Rather, it's about re-figuring out how to eat outside of the eating regimen mindset, putting the emphasis on your personal signs (otherwise known as your instinct) like craving, totality, and fulfilment, and moving ceaselessly from outer prompts like nourishment rules and confinements.

However, intuitive eating isn't the 'hunger-totality diet.' Intuitive eaters give themselves unrestricted consent to eat anything they desire without feeling regretful. They depend on their inner craving and satiety flag and trust their body to disclose to them what, when, and the amount to eat. They know when they need to eat veggies and when they want to have dessert (and don't feel remorseful or have any second thoughts with either decision).

There aren't any principles!

I'm going to be level with you: slimming down is more uncomplicated than intuitive eating. Why? Because there is a set measure of rules to pursue, and it's extremely clear. Try not to eat this. Simply eat that. Anticipate this outcome in 21 days. That is basically what an eating routine is.

Intuitive eating is progressively about INTERNAL heavy work.

What's more, there aren't firm rules. It appears to be unique for everybody (and that is the point).

Here is an account of an intuitive eater; something changed in me eighteen months in the wake of graduating school.

It was about a similar time when I understood I never again needed to seek after a profession in media outlets.

I understood looking great, as indicated by all standards, didn't generally make a difference. Looking "hot" didn't make me a superior human. Restricting diets didn't cause me to make an incredible more.

Essentially, I understood life is too short to even consider caring SO MUCH about my appearance and that certainty originates from inside.

I quit wearing a lot of cosmetics. I quit going through $400/month on garments I didn't wear. Furthermore, I quit annihilating myself indulging in two cuts of pizza.

I loosen myself. Furthermore, don't think I surrendered.

My intuitive eating story is not the same as the others that I've perused. The vast majority of the tales include a stage where a previous calorie counter eats whatever she wants for a considerable length of time until understanding that her body really hungers for healthy nourishments.

I generally ate unhealthy nourishments. In any event, when counting calories. I'm certain you have as well.

The move for me was taking the concentration off calories and parcels and on setting aside cash for doing stuff I thought about.

I began cooking, and I sort of realized that on the off chance that I was making it myself at home, I couldn't feel regretful about it. Regardless of whether it was something I some time ago thought to be "unhealthy."

At the point when I began cooking, I quit thinking about the "great" and "terrible" part of nutrition and began thinking about if what I was eating made me feel fulfilled without needing to sleep after lunch.

I was effectively trying various suppers, scanning for what made me feel stimulated and fulfilled without any blame or misery or lament.

Meal prep and cooking helped me reconnect with my nourishment and my body. What's more, following a half year of preparing 70% of my suppers and ENJOYING foods I ate out at cafés (rather than feeling remorseful about it), my body has continued as before size (a size I'm so alright with) for a long time. Nothing should be fixed. I do not expect to attempt to change my body any longer.

It comes down to TRUST.

Intuitive eating isn't tied in with eating anything you desire; it's tied in with eating what your body needs and having the option to focus on that WITHOUT your mind disrupting the general flow to scrutinize your choices.

Now and then, your body needs an enormous bowl of veggies. Once in a while, it needs pizza and sushi.

What's more, when you enable yourself to have anything you need, the previous defiant intrigue of low-quality nourishment vanishes since you can have it whenever.

Furthermore, when you free your psyche from all the eating regimen BS that has been latched onto your subconscious mind for quite a long time, you'll see that you can utilize that valuable mental ability for different things.

Like redesigning your profession.

Being a superior parent/ partner/ companion.

Grabbing another leisure activity. Or on the other hand, beginning a business.

For me, intuitive eating has a fabulous time as opposed to something to fear. Also, that is the thing that I need you to feel too. I need you to feel positive about your nourishment decisions and realize that they're YOUR business as it were. You get the opportunity to make up the standards.

Chapter 2: Dieter's headache

In 2016, Molly Bahr changed as long as she can remember with a Google search. Bahr, a specialist, was at an expert training program on dietary problems when a speaker referenced in passing that members may be keen on something many refer to as intuitive eating. Bahr looked into the term. "I returned home that day, and it resembled a light switch," she says. "I had a feeling that I got hit by a truck."

Bahr concluded that she needed to get the message out about intuitive eating, yet there was one issue. Up to that minute, she had been devoted to customary thoughts of abstaining from excessive food intake and wellbeing, empowering devotees of her developing wellness-centred Instagram record to gauge their nourishment, watch their dietary macros, and fuss over their weight as an essential marker of their wellbeing. Intuitive eating, then again, is a hypothesis that places the inverse: Calorie checking, carb evading, and waistline estimating are making individuals sincerely hopeless, however adding to huge numbers of the medical issues recently credited to basic indulging.

Bahr says intuitive eating changed both how she treated her patients and what she looked like at herself. She had been continually gauging and shooting herself, attempting to hit objectives that she says were separated from how she really felt. "It was challenging for me to understand that I had been so cruel to my very own body, despite the fact that in my mind, I was doing it for wellbeing," she says. Changing the direction of her open Instagram record was ungainly; however, she had a feeling that she should have been straightforward with individuals. "One day I needed to think of a post that resembled, 'Hello, sorry for all that I've at any point said. It was, in reality, all off-base,'" she says.

Presently Bahr posts messages in a style that has turned out to be increasingly normal in the previous year: plain content on an everyday foundation, with suggestions to focus on your physical sentiments of appetite or to cast away blame overeating well-loved nourishment. In doing that, she has turned out to be one of a developing number of specialists, dietitians, and nutritionists who have increased a dedicated after on Instagram in view of intuitive eating. These experts urge adherents to chip away at their association with nourishment without agonizing over their weight and to dismiss the thoughts of temperance and sin that have supported social beliefs regarding eating since days of yore.

As these records accumulate a huge number of supporters and attempt to beat back the absolute most hurtful thoughts of Instagram's military of novice health specialists, they seem to have taken advantage of the developing dissatisfactions that numerous individuals—and most ladies—have with slimming down. Americans are tired of the disgrace and dread surrounding diet and of disappointment before the close unconquerable chances of long-haul weight reduction. Shouldn't there be a preferred way?

Albeit intuitive eating's on the web ubiquity is extending, the idea has been around for two or three decades. In 1995, Evelyn Tribole and Elyse Resch, a couple of dietitians in Southern California, distributed their first book on this same topic after watching their customers do what a great part of the accessible research says is practically inescapable: recapture weight that had been lost while consuming fewer calories. They had been utilizing a similar methodology that fundamentally all dietitians pursued in those days, which held that body weight was of essential significance in assessing and improving dietary wellbeing. "We were striking our heads against the divider on the grounds that the manner in which we were working wasn't working,"

Numerous dietitians still depend on this methodology as a result of heftiness's relationship with conditions, for example, coronary illness and diabetes, and the thriving notoriety of intuitive eating has made something of a part in the field. It is accepted that deprioritizing weight for different markers of prosperity can have a significantly valuable impact on individuals' wellbeing all its own. Frequently, individuals who neglect to get more fit and the individuals who restore it are thought to be sluggish or too uneducated even to consider making great decisions. That couldn't possibly be more off-base in her experience. "Our patients are truly successful and smart individuals, else," she says. And keeping in mind that the cycle of weight reduction and increase is unhealthy all alone, the emotional disgrace appended to it causes another round of harm.

Intuitive eating was created to address both of these tricky layers in eating less junk food. They urge individuals to accomplish something that may sound clamorous or perilous: Eat what you need, without any standards about what to eat, its amount, or when. Intuitive eating has ten principles(which will be discussed later in the book); however, the most notable one is that no nourishments are forbidden and that there is nothing of the sort as a "decent" or "terrible" nourishment.

That is in an apparent restriction to another school of nourishment felt that is picked up notoriety on

Instagram: clean eating. In case you eat clean, you have to give careful consideration to any nourishment's place on a continuum of virtue, and eat just the things that fulfil the strictest guidelines of natural freshness. Eating today has turned into this thought; the nourishment on your fork can either kill you or fix you. It's arrived at a point of practically strict enthusiasm.

By correlation, intuitive eating seems like consent to sit on your lounge chair and eat pizza until you go out. In any case, Tribole and Bahr don't deny that various nourishments have distinctive dietary advantages, or intend to tear down general wellbeing activities that advise children to eat vegetables. Rather, they state they need to help individuals who have battled with eating see how nourishment makes their body feel when the demonstration is unravelled from pressure or disgrace. Both Tribole and Bahr find that in the initial week or two, new followers of intuitive eating do here, and there gorge on the things they had constantly attempted to skip. Be that as it may, the two analysts state by far most of their customers rapidly habituate to burgers or doughnuts and afterward hunger for the assortment and nourishment spoke to by the "sound" food sources they once utilized as a discipline.

The hypothesis is that in the event that you can have pizza at whatever point you need, it feels less fundamental to eat it until you're awkward when the open door presents itself, or to search out the open door by any means. Revealing to yourself you can't have something, in the meantime, gives it undue power and charm. "I didn't comprehend that the gorges were made from the limitation," Bahr says. "I thought I was a creature." previously, look into has demonstrated that American ladies disguise the significance of confining nourishment consumption as youthful as age 5, making it practically difficult to test how individuals would act toward nourishment on the off chance that they weren't shackled by a culture of abstaining from excessive food intake. It is frequently considered the unnatural inclination to eat specific nourishment that emerges on account of foreseen limitation the "last-dinner impact." "It's the consent oddity," she says. "At the point when you have consent to eat, the nourishment still tastes great, yet you expel the desperation."

That sentiment of desperation is likely natural to a great many people, regardless of whether they generally thought of the need to cling to some sort of nourishment administers as absolutely typical and sound. In spite of the fact that the quantity of individuals who may search out the administrations of a dietitian is moderately little, the group of spectators who could profit by better approaches for seeing nourishment is a lot bigger. As per a 2008 study by the University of North Carolina at Chapel Hill, 75 percent of American ladies partake in some sort of cluttered eating conduct, regardless of whether their issues aren't extreme enough to comprise a clinical finding of a dietary problem.

Recommending that a stable association with nutrition is conceivable with no standards or limitations sounds dangerous to numerous individuals, particularly when it's confused as a call to enjoy ruinous motivations instead of to comprehend and calm them. Intuitive eating has an alluring sound of simplicity and change that is utilized for advertising numerous sorts of diets. That has likely helped it burst into flames via web-based networking media, where comparable messages of energy and future joy are utilized to sell a wide range of restrictive eating practices and craving suppressants. Not at all like how health slants, as a rule, happen on Instagram, however, the idea's designers aren't behind its open push, and they don't have a lot to sell you. "I began Instagram like three months back. I had no clue that my kin are there. I thought it was a Kardashian thing, so I was extremely hesitant to try and jump on."

In that manner, intuitive eating is just about as grassroots as a nourishment philosophy can get. You can find out about it online for nothing, including the majority of the significant rules that make it conceivable to rehearse without anyone else. There are no feast designs, no healthy shakes, no marked nourishment stockpiling frameworks, no solidified suppers in your market. At last, the objective is to quit paying the experts who may have acquainted you with the thought. When you get it, you get it. You don't need to do treatment and meet with a dietitian for a mind-blowing remainder.

This shouldn't imply that that intuitive eating is an ensured approach to get thinner or fix whatever you believe is physically amiss with you. In the event that any health expert or mentor or Instagram influencer says you can get more fit with intuitive eating, flee. Nobody can disclose to you what will happen to your body. Everything relies upon where you, as of now, are comparative with your body's regular weight, which may or probably won't coordinate with customary ideas of what a "solid" weight would be for your tallness.

Fundamental examinations have discovered intuitive eating less viable for momentary weight reduction than customarily prohibitive eating regimens. In any case, examine has additionally discovered that it can improve self-perception in young ladies and that care practices, for example, contemplation, which (like intuitive eating) are planned to all the more likely adjust individuals to their bodies, are successful approaches to intervene gorge and passionate eating propensities.

Like Bahr, a possibility experience with intuitive eating likewise set Sami Main's life a totally different way, yet hers was through the sort of Instagram multiplication that Bahr has helped gotten underway. Fundamental, a writer, ran over a rundown of Instagram dietitians worth after and got inquisitive. "I began following a portion of those records, and they all appeared to be so certain in such an abnormal way, that health Instagram doesn't generally hit," she says. At the time, Main had been in recuperation for a dietary problem for a couple of years, and the inspiration addressed her. "Getting more fit doesn't really make you more advantageous, as a wide assortment of dietary problems can let you know," she says.

Subsequent to getting familiar with intuitive eating and standing out the methodology from how specialists had taken care of her dietary problem, Main chose to return to class to turn into a dietitian. "A portion of the prepared medicinal specialists that I saw, including a nutritionist and a gastroenterologist, didn't get my dietary issue and weren't at all readied to offer guidance on it," she says. Slimming down and nourishment limitation are such imbued pieces of American culture that even specialists can experience considerable difficulties outlining among sound and destructive practices, which is the place intuitive eating's potential power falsehoods, and why Main felt attracted to change her calling.

James Greenblatt, a specialist who has worked with a considerable number of patients with dietary issues, urges a mindful way to deal with intuitive eating for those battling intensely with nourishment. "I worry that an excessive number of patients that I've seen who had genuine dietary issues were being treated with a careful or instinctive methodology, and it wasn't fruitful," he says. A few people can't appropriately control their nourishment consumption on a natural level, and for those individuals, another mentality just postpones powerful treatment. "To me, [intuitive eating] is frequently the subsequent advance," Greenblatt proceeds. "The initial step is to get the science levelled out, and at times that is a drug."

In spite of his reservations, Greenblatt says that the vast majority of the standards behind intuitive eating are consistent and that they're significant in attempting to battle the disgrace numerous individuals have around eating, which, in his experience, is stirred by Instagram specifically. "Online networking has truly been terrible, particularly for our preteen young ladies, and it's a detour to individuals looking for help or recognizing that they may have an issue," he says.

In that limit, the multiplication of intuitive eating records and images can, in any event, give an antithesis to the endless support to go on a juice purify or look for noticeable abs. Bahr says that she's likewise observed intuitive eating help her patients with uneasiness and discouragement by urging them to appreciate things and be social. "You understand how little your life has moved toward becoming when you're abstaining from excessive food intake," she says. Individuals on abstains from food regularly dread or maintain a strategic distance from social circumstances on the grounds that those often include calories, which can be segregating and push individuals over the line into dietary issues.

The American culture around nourishment and eating may be arriving at an emphasis. Numerous dietitians still lecture conventional weight-based models, yet research is beginning to heap up in manners that demonstrate those individuals may be feeling the loss of the backwoods for the trees. For instance, the all overweight cycling that is basic among calorie counters may really be more hurtful to an individual's wellbeing than never losing the weight regardless, and the disgrace against chunky individuals that abstaining from excessive food intake supports may be liable for a portion of the wellbeing hurts recently connected to obesity itself.

The deep-rooted strain to eat fewer carbs wears individuals out. It's obvious that a few clinicians and calorie counters in the long run search for another way—however, it may be increasingly exact to consider intuitive eating an old way. "We were altogether brought into the world as instinctive eaters," Bahr says. "I love viewing my nieces and nephews eat. They generally know when they need to stop."

Chapter 3: Thinking like an intuitive eater

Consistently, we're immersed with new diet drifts and refreshed dietary guidance. Dietitians, specialists, and self-educated specialists yell more than each other: eat clean, quit eating gluten, attempt Whole30, or eat like a cave dweller. It's close to difficult to make an educated, empowering choice amid the clashing messages. One methodology that is transcending the conflict requests that you hurl out tried and true ways of thinking — dismiss the eating routine attitude! — and grasp intuitive eating. The idea may be more recognizable than you might suspect.

Intuitive eating frequently alluded to as a "hostile to eat fewer carbs," sounds confounded; however, it just means tuning in to your body, confiding in your gut (actually), and doing what makes you feel better. Rather than tallying calories, you quit eating when you feel full. Rather than "eating your sentiments," you "regard your body." Instead of "good" or "awful" nourishments, you have the opportunity to eat whatever you want. At the point when you feel that empty inclination or protesting in your stomach, you ought to react with what your body wants.

At whatever point I'm conversing with somebody about intuitive eating just because I generally stress that it's an adventure that requires some investment. It's absolutely not something that occurs without any forethought; it requires exertion. It might be disappointing en route, since we are so engrained in diet culture nowadays, which is the reason I firmly propose working with an enlisted dietitian who spends significant time in intuitive eating.

As a boost, intuitive eating is a non-diet way to deal with eating. It is a feasible method for eating that is free of rules and confinements. It's tied in with figuring out how to tune in to and comprehend your body, figuring out how to support it in the most ideal manner conceivable while fulfilling both your needs and needs. It's tied in with building up a positive association with nourishment. All impressive stuff, isn't that so? I suspect as much as well.

Intuitive eating has sincerely been extraordinary for me. I'm open about my multi-year battle with a dietary issue, which was the darkest a great time. Much after my weight settled, I battled with eating less junk food, feeling that I needed to eat a specific path so as to eat "sound." Nourishment expended my musings. When might I eat? What might I eat?

Furthermore, God forbid I need to go OUT to eat! That was the most exceedingly awful, not being responsible for each part of nourishment. It wasn't until I discovered intuitive eating that my association with nourishment genuinely improved.

I don't intend to discuss intuitive eating like it is this All-Mighty being or anything. Truth be told, it's idiotic straightforward. It's typical eating. In any case, I find that this effortlessness has gotten SO lost in diet culture.

It is the point at which you tune in to your body and eat what makes YOU feel better. You restore this common confidence with yourself that may have gotten lost someplace in the years that we were presented to the counting calories world. The beneficial thing is, with training, we can prepare ourselves again to eat when we're hungry normally and normally stop when we are fulfilled/full. Much the same as an infant who might cry when they need breastmilk and a multi-year old who wouldn't like to complete her plate since she genuinely is full! No diet is custom like a natural one! Furthermore, as insane as it might appear, when you quit concentrating such a considerable amount on eating less, you'll really eat less. My objective right now is to assist individuals with recuperating the eating fewer carbs brain and more towards an increasingly legitimate association with nourishment. I used to eat in light of the fact that it was the ideal opportunity for a specific feast or on the grounds that I returned home, and I would experience the kitchen. At the point when this occurred, I constantly ended up feeling full, enlarged, not ravenous at supper time, and by and large, disappointed with nourishment and the manner in which my body was beginning to look. Presently, I eat when I'm eager, and I stop when I'm full. More difficult than one might expect... I know. Be that as it may, when you start following the means (underneath), you will turn out to be more in contact with your body and begin to confide in it. I presently acknowledge how fulfilling nourishment truly is the point at which I am genuinely starved, and I likewise acknowledge how great my body feels when regarding my totality.

You're backing off and tuning in while you eat - really tasting your nourishment! You've begun to get reacquainted with the unobtrusive moves by the way you feel as your stomach fills and exhausts as opposed to holding back to eat until you're excruciatingly eager to eat, and afterward holding off on halting until you're insufferably full.

But then...

At the point when you see your pants feeling cozy, you quickly second guess all that you ate in the course of the most recent 48 hours, notwithstanding the way that it was scrumptious, satisfied you, and you felt really great while eating it and a while later. You end up enticed to haul the scale-out of the storage room just to check and ensure it swells from that Mexican wrap you had for lunch, and that you're not putting on weight. The following day you pack a sub-par plate of mixed greens for lunch, attempting to be "great," just to wind up thoughtlessly crunching on the treat bowl throughout the evening. Eager and tired at supper that night, you eat past the purpose of agreeable fulfilment and wind up feeling stuffed. You lay wakeful in bed that late evening, pondering, "will I ever be an intuitive eater? Possibly I'm too broken even to consider making harmony with nourishment."

You're taking every necessary step. You see the promising finish to the present course of action. In any case, how much longer until you at last feel like nourishment and eating isn't so upsetting. To what extent until I become an intuitive eater?

I wish there were a simple answer, yet it's SO individual from individual to individual. For one customer, essentially, my giving verbal authorization to eat carbs and sugar was sufficient to get off the confine/gorge cycle. It's scarcely ever that simple. For most, making harmony with nourishment is an adventure of numerous years. In case you're finding that it's taking that long, realize that there's nothing amiss with you. On the off chance that you've been consuming fewer calories or limiting for most your life, at that point, it might enjoy a long time to delay those old neural pathways driving prohibitive and gorging practices around nourishment.

Additionally, remember, there is no "official" natural eater. Being an intuitive eater is certainly not a dark or white definition. There's no test you can pass or declaration you're granted or permit you to gain. It's additionally extremely typical for natural eaters to settle on choices that aren't so instinctive once in a while, or to incidentally fall once more into old prohibitive practices when encountering a real existence change. It might seem like a figure of speech; however, intuitive eating genuinely is an adventure and not a goal.

Here's the memory of a nursing mother; I don't care for "diet." I don't care for limitations. I don't care for setting myself up for disappointment. A few days, I wake up, and I'm starving, so I have a huge breakfast. Different days, I have no craving, so I drink my frosted espresso, get a bunch of almonds, and go on with my day until the little food cravings settle in. It took me decades to figure out how to be an intuitive eater. In any case, two healthy pregnancies (and kids) later, I can genuinely say I did it. What's more, I have a three-year-old to thank for it.

Allow me to clarify.

At the point when you're a lady, your companions, family, and associates have huge amounts of feelings about what you resemble. At the point when you're a nutritionist, their assessments and presumptions at that point lead to inquiries regarding what you do and don't eat. Sharing a supper consistently prompts an examination. "Do you eat dairy?" "Have you at any point gone, Paleo?" "Is sugar hazardous?"

My little child hasn't heard anything about this. Truth be told, he just eats when he's ravenous. He won't eat when he's full, and he possibly tidbits when he needs a little burst of vitality to get him through until his next feast.

From the outset, I moved toward the majority of this as an issue that required tackling. I gave putting him a shot a calendar: feeding him breakfast inside thirty minutes of waking, followed by a hearty lunch an hour prior to his rest, etc. At the point when he would not eat, I counselled with his paediatrician. All things considered, how could the child of a wellbeing expert be supplement inadequate?

In any case, here's the intelligent thing: It turns out he was getting what he required.

He was tuning in to his body. Actually, he was more on top of his caloric needs than the greater part of us are. Being a little child, my child doesn't get that, by American principles, breakfast is the most significant supper of the day. He couldn't care less that most wellbeing specialists teach you to quit eating a few hours before you hit the sack. He never discovered that drinking an eight-ounce glass of water before a feast will check your craving. He's three, and he couldn't care less. He tunes in to his body, and he eats when his little belly instructs him to.

I understood that was something I could truly gain from.

Truly, we invest an excessive amount of energy fixating on our "abstains from food." We name what kind of eaters we are and what sorts of eating will cause us to get in shape, or beef up, or feel our best. It would be unfair of me to state that I never attempted to remove complex carbs, sugar, caffeine, or different nourishments named "awful" sooner or later in my life. It's hard to tell how our bodies react to devouring certain nourishments, and it might bode well for you to attempt to kill them every once in a while.

However, the sooner we acknowledge the way that there is no enchantment way—no enchantment "fix"— the sooner we can get back in line with what our bodies long for and make fair, more advantageous nourishment decisions. Hello, three-year-olds appear to have a ton of fun than we are, isn't that so?

Here are five stages prescribed to become an Intuitive eater:

1. Understand that planning isn't all that matters.

Quit utilizing a clock to choose when to eat. Breakfast is significant, yet whether you eat it at 6:00 a.m. or on the other hand, 9:00 a.m. won't represent the deciding moment your day.

2. Change your point of view.

At the point when we go on "consumes fewer calories," one bunch of M&M's misleads us. We all of a sudden think we've fizzled, and we go from feeling roused to feeling crushed in less than ten seconds. Try not to search for momentary arrangements; consider the master plan.

3. Keep in mind calories are not the villain.

Huge numbers of us exercise to consume off the majority of the nourishment we ate. We overlook that calories give us.

4. Bet everything.

In case you need French fries, don't make do with pretzels. Eating something other than what's expected won't avert the hankering, and you'll wind up eating both the pretzels and the French fries. Simply focus on those yearnings and attempt to make sense of what's making them keep them from springing up once more.

5. Eat one meal at a time.

Try not to think about every day as a "decent" or "terrible" day dependent on what you ate. Reset your clock at every feast. Along these lines, if your morning meal is waffles, you aren't in the outlook of, "Today I ate inadequately, I'll start again tomorrow."

As the periods of life change, so does your association with nourishment. You may arrive at a point where you think about yourself an intuitive eater; at that point, get determined to have an ailment that requires changing your dietary patterns. Experiencing a progress period as you figure out how to deal with your body in another manner is not out of the ordinary. Life may change to where you possess less energy for self-consideration - ventures at work, extend at home, having children, a disease in the family, taking on a volunteer job, returning to class, and so on. In these circumstances, you'll likely be less careful around nourishment, and thus less in line with your body's needs, and perhaps commit a couple of errors in eating. It's alright.

Eating practices are profoundly entwined with self-perception, so changes in mentalities towards your body will definitely influence your association with nourishment. What's more, with regards to body acknowledgement, it's never a done arrangement. As you experience life, your body will change. You may attempt to battle it, take a gander at any multi-year old beside a multi-year old, and we can realize that this will generally be valid. The way toward tolerating your body is never done on the grounds that your body is always showing signs of change.

In case you're feeling stuck or disappointed with your intuitive eating venture, if it's not too much trouble, realize that what you're doing is difficult - extremely hard! You're conflicting with forever and a day of informing you've retained from diet culture, and doing something contrary to what you've generally been advised to do - confine and control nourishment. Do whatever it takes not to pass judgment on yourself on some envisioned result, as it is an interruption from the learning and development you've just cultivated.

Chapter 4: Know the kind of eater you are

Have you at any point really thought about to what sort of eater you are? All things considered, much like design, everybody has their very own style with regards to dietary patterns. Diet, recurrence, and sentiments of completion and starvation the same all show distinctively in individuals. And keeping in mind that deciding your own eating type may sound plain as day, it's, in reality, more intricate than you may suspect.

Do any of these circumstances sound natural?

- Your suppers typically leave a container, a vacuum-gathered sack, or over the shop counter.

- You never eat alone: TV, the Internet, telephone, or your preferred magazine is there for almost every dinner.

- You discover it beside difficult to leave free nourishment, regardless of whether you're not eager – including everything you-can-eat buffets, general store test tables, and those "taste me" stalls at swap meets.

- You invest more energy lamenting what you ate than setting it up.

- You eat when you're ravenous. Additionally, when you're tragic, distraught, hurt, irritated, disturbed – even, in some cases, when you're excited.

On the off chance that you end up saying, "That is me," you may have fallen prey to at least one undesirable eating style, supper time, or way of life propensities that can hinder weight control.

Here and there, dangerous eating examples are anything but difficult to spot, for example, when you go to nourishment each time you're confronting an issue. In any case, frequently, the prompts are inconspicuous to the point that these undesirable propensities go unnoticed.

There are six unique sorts of eating styles, each with their very own arrangement of practices and propensities. Here, we convey our knowledge, alongside tips on how you can battle everyone.

1. Emotional eater

Is it accurate to say that you are an emotional eater?

In case you're an individual who snatches 16 ounces of Ben and all Jerry's occasions you've had a terrible day at work, you're probably an emotional eater. This kind of eater depicts an individual who expends calories to celebrate when they're glad or sulks when they're dismal. Basically, what, how, and when you eat all returns to how you feel. There's no pondering how what you're eating will make you feel sooner rather than later; an enthusiastic eater essentially hopes to fulfil a feeling with nourishment dependent on a given minute.

2. Habitual eater

Supper arranging can support ongoing eaters.

Somebody who regularly enjoys terrible nourishment under the "simply this once" pardon is a routine eater. Despite the fact that they like daily schedule and structure, and they realize how to eat right and exercise consistently, ongoing eaters are regularly crashed by time limitations and obligations. Moreover, these sorts of individuals frequently eat in any event, when they're not eager, mostly because they are accustomed to doing it. The issue with ongoing eating is that it shields you from burning some major calories and eating on plan.

3. External eater

Oreos may make you need to eat in case you're an outside eater.

External eaters are an advertiser's fantasy: Food publicizing, seeing a birthday cake in the workplace, and such fill in as outer prompts that trigger an individual to eat. Seeing cupcakes in a presentation window or engaging eatery contributions can, without much of a stretch, spark your mind into speculation you have to eat, in any event, when you don't. All the outside components that address you by and by indicate the weight or want to gorge.

4. Critical eater

Basic eaters can wind up over the top.

This is the "win big or bust" kind of individual. A basic eater knows the significance of nourishment, yet their commitment to slimming down is over the top. Be that as it may, a basic eater can likewise experience serious difficulties adhering to a reliably solid eating routine. They're either on the rails, or they're off. When on an eating routine, basic eaters see themselves as "great," yet when off, they're "terrible." They can without much of a stretch skip from eating a whole box of low-fat treats, to convenient solution diets like squeezing.

5. Sensual eater

Be careful with a wanton buffet.

In case you're somebody who genuinely acknowledges nourishment and appreciates each and every chomp, you can place yourself into the sexy eater classification. You're not one to race through dinner, and for what reason would it be advisable for you too? You very much want to savour the exploration and scrumptiousness of new nourishment than comply with the limitations of a demanding eater. You'll have a go at anything once, and you likely have a couple of additional pounds to bear since you discover more delight in eating than you do in dependable, nourishment related basic leadership.

6. Energy eater

Energy eaters may eat an excessive number of tidbits.

You'd most likely accept this one has a lot to do with those searching for a speedy vitality fix, and you'd be correct. Energy eaters centre around solid, in a hurry snacks, however to the outrageous, regularly eating such a large number of them. While solid nibbling is incredible, depending too vigorously on it tends to be counterproductive for your general wellbeing objectives. While it's essential to tune in to your craving and eat quick-acting sugars, similar to bread, saltines, and granola bars, when you have to, you could be expending a more significant number of calories than your body requires, while additionally expanding your insulin creation. At last, this can cause more appetite.

Chapter 5: Separating emotions & hunger

What causes somebody to go from just being starved to all-out "hangry"? Something other than a straightforward drop in glucose, this mix of appetite and outrage might be an entangled emotional reaction, including a transaction of science, character, and ecological signs.

Improve or calm pressure? These tips can assist you with halting enthusiastic eating, battle yearnings, recognize your triggers, and discover additionally fulfilling approaches to encourage your emotions.

We don't generally eat just to fulfil a physical craving. A considerable lot of us likewise go to nourishment for comfort, stress help, or to compensate ourselves. Furthermore, when we do, we will, in general, reach for shoddy food, desserts, and other encouraging yet unhealthy nourishments. You may go after 16 ounces of frozen yoghurt when you're feeling down, request a pizza in case you're exhausted or forlorn, or swing by the drive-through following a distressing day at work. Passionate eating is utilizing nourishment to make yourself feel good—to fill enthusiastic needs, as opposed to your stomach. Shockingly, emotional eating doesn't fix emotional issues. Indeed, it more often than not exacerbates you feel. A short time later, not exclusively does the first intense subject matter remain; however, you additionally feel remorseful for gorging.

Once in a while, utilizing nourishment as a stimulating beverage, a reward, or to celebrate isn't really a terrible thing. Be that as it may, when eating is your essential emotional method for dealing with stress—when your first motivation is to open the icebox at whatever point you're focused on, resentful, furious, forlorn, depleted, or exhausted—you stall out in an undesirable cycle where the genuine inclination or issue is rarely tended to.

Emotional yearning can't be loaded up with nourishment. Eating may feel great at the time;

however, the emotions that set off the consumption are still there. What's more, you regularly feel more awful than you did before due to the excessive calories you've quite recently devoured. You beat yourself for failing and not having more self-control.

Intensifying the issue, you quit learning more advantageous approaches to manage your feelings, you have an increasingly hard time controlling your weight, and you feel progressively feeble over both nourishment and your emotions. However, regardless of how ineffective you feel over food and your sentiments, it is conceivable to roll out an improvement. You can learn more advantageous approaches to manage your feelings, keep away from triggers, overcome longings, lastly, put a stop to emotional eating.

The distinction between emotional and physical eating;

Before you can break free from the cycle of emotional eating, you first need to figure out how to recognize emotional and physical appetite. This can be trickier than it sounds, particularly on the off chance that you routinely use nourishment to manage your sentiments.

Emotional appetite can be incredible, so it's anything but difficult to confuse it with physical eating. Be that as it may, there are pieces of information you can search for to assist you with distinguishing physical and emotional eating.

Emotional eating goes ahead all of a sudden. It hits you in a moment and feels overpowering and critical. Physical eating, then again, goes ahead more step by step. The desire to eat doesn't feel as desperate or request moment fulfilment (except if you haven't eaten for quite a while).

Emotional eating needs explicit solace nourishments. At the point when you're physically ravenous, nearly anything sounds great—including solid stuff like vegetables. Yet, emotional eating hungers for lousy nourishment or sugary tidbits that give a moment surge. You have an inclination that you need cheesecake or pizza, and everything else should be ignored.

Emotional eating frequently prompts thoughtless eating. Before you know it, you've eaten an entire pack of chips or a whole 16 ounces of frozen yoghurt without truly focusing or completely getting a charge out of it. At the point when you're eating because of physical eating, you're regularly mindful of what you're doing.

Emotional craving isn't fulfilled once you're full. You continue the need to an ever-increasing extent, frequently eating until you're awkwardly stuffed. Physical desire, then again, shouldn't be complete. You feel fulfilled when your stomach is full.

An emotional appetite isn't situated in the stomach. As opposed to a snarling midsection or an ache in your stomach, you feel your yearning as a hankering you can't escape your head. You're focussed around explicit surfaces, tastes, and scents.

Emotional appetite frequently prompts lament, blame, or disgrace. At the point when you eat to fulfil physical yearning, you're probably not going to feel regretful or embarrassed in light of the fact that you're essentially giving your body what it needs. In the event that you feel remorseful after you eat, it's feasible on the grounds that you realize where it counts that you're not eating for hygienic reasons.

Intuitive eating is additionally about figuring out how to perceive the input from your body about the nourishment you eat, so you can settle on decisions that work for your body (and wellbeing) just as your taste buds. Be that as it may, it's not just about the body – Intuitive Eating includes dealing with your psyche as well – in such a case that you've been abstaining from excessive food intake for a considerable length of time, you'll have disguised the Diet Police – rules got or made up, about what, when and the amount to eat and work out; just as cruel reactions about your body and how you should look… every one of these messages should be perceived and tested.

What is Mindful Eating?

Mindfulness is an act of staying alert right now, without judgment. It's basically about awareness and acceptance. In case you're focusing on your present eating background, you'll know about:

- your thoughts (about the nourishment, your body, or in truth whatever else)
- your physical sentiments
- your emotional emotions
- your starvation level
- your purpose of fulfilment
- the taste of the nourishment
- the smell of it
- how it looks

You can overeat and still be careful. You can also binge and be mindful of it. The thing that matters is that you're doing it with mindfulness. What's more, when you have mindfulness, your decisions open up to you. At the point when your mindfulness is missing, and you're on autopilot, at that point, choices don't appear to be that accessible.

The advantages of eating carefully and instinctively

In the event that you choose to oust slims down from your life, and grasp natural and careful eating, you won't think back.

No more blame!

At the point when you genuinely give yourself unrestricted authorization to eat what you need, when you need, your yearnings will fundamentally decrease – and will be all the more physically based, as opposed to as a response to confinement or hardship.

No more crazies!

You won't consider nourishment from the time you open your eyes toward the beginning of the day to the time you close them again around evening time. You'll wake up with different things to consider, not whether you'll fit into your garments today, or scolding yourself for how you ate yesterday – or stressed over how you'll eat today.

You'll consider nourishment generally when you're eager, or when you have to do the shopping for food. Periodically on different occasions, your consideration will be gotten by musings of nourishment; however, you'll have enough practice and involvement with seeing the idea and releasing it for it not to be anything over transitory.

Also, when you do once in a while eat for reasons other than hunger, you'll let it go, similar to a hot potato since you'll realize that everybody indulges once in a while — no major ordeal. You'll proceed onward rapidly, and eat again when you're next hungry.

No additionally gorging!

Would you be able to see that when you're not prohibiting any nourishments, not going hungry, not limiting or checking – but instead, eating an assortment of food sources with some restraint, as per your yearning and fulfillment signals, and tolerating yourself as you seem to be, that you will at any rate, profoundly lessen, and likely quit gorging by and large?

Give your body a chance to locate its upbeat weight

With the steady practice of intuitive and mindful eating, your body will locate its common, glad weight. That is a weight that doesn't take unreasonable measures of vitality and mental concentration to continue. It's a weight that enables you to feel settled both with nourishment and your body. It may not be the body you had always wanted, yet let's face it – your body disappointment is very likely in light of disguised social magnificence models – so maybe it's not the body you had always wanted – but rather the body of culture's interest, which for practically we all are either difficult to accomplish (because of hereditary qualities) or requires over the top thoughtfulness regarding what, when and the amount to eat; and what, when and the amount to work out.

Energy for different things

With less vitality consumed on contemplating your body, weight, and nourishment, you'll be opened up to make, take part in, and appreciate life! I simply completed the process of talking with a customer this evening, who said, 'without this, I realize I can go far in my profession.' She perceives the obstruction of over the top, considering her body and nourishment, on her capacity to contribute genuinely to society. Furthermore, she needs more for her life.

Greater happiness

As you unravel yourself from the hold of a diet mindset, you'll discover greater pleasure throughout everyday life. Rather than causing yourself to go to the rec center to do a hard exercise, when you're hounding tired, you may pick a hot shower, or a yoga class – or going out to see a film with a companion. You may take a gander at a café menu with a genuine interest in the alternatives, instead of search for the choice with the least carbs or calories.

You'll slack off.

Become increasingly adaptable in your reasoning and conduct.

THE QUALITY OF YOUR WHOLE LIFE WILL IMPROVE.

Not simply your psychological and physical wellbeing.

On the off chance that you've been rehearsing natural and careful eating – what different advantages have you encountered? Tell me in the remarks. I'd love to know about your encounters.

How To Stop Emotional Eating?

The fundamental method to stop emotional eating is to distinguish what you truly need to assist you with adapting to that particular inclination. Next time you experience one of these feelings, take a stab at doing one of these exercises as opposed to eating.

On the off chance that you feel Tired or Restless:

- Taking a rest
- Enjoying a bubble shower
- Listening to music
- Meditate or take a couple of full breaths
- Stretch

In the event that you feel Frustrated or Misunderstood:

- Call a companion
- Write in your diary
- Write a litter
- Comfort the circumstance

In the event that you feel Sad, Lonely, or Discouraged:

- Meet a companion or relative for espresso
- Join a local gathering
- Call a relative

- Get moving – endorphins is an incredible state of mind booster

In the event that you feel Bored, Angry, or Anxious:

- Get some outside air
- Dance to your preferred tunes
- Chat with a companion or relative
- Work on an interest

By managing your passionate triggers in profitable manners, you will step by step decrease the propensity for depending on nourishment to soothe your sentiments, and you may see an immediate effect on your waistline! It is additionally critical to adhere to your sketched-out dinner plan as intently as could reasonably be expected, regardless of how you are feeling that day. On the off chance that you wind up skirting a feast or missing your evening nibble, there is a decent possibility you will move toward becoming "hangry," which will just further your passionate shakiness. Keep this from occurring by ensuring you are firmly following your sketched-out diet plan.

Whatever feelings you are feeling, channel that vitality into physical movement! Exercise is an effective option to utilize when you are feeling any kind of emotional shakiness. In addition to the fact that it aids in your weight reduction venture, but at the same time, it's an extraordinary method to diminish pressure and tension. A great many people realize that moving more is useful for your heart — yet scarcely any know it's additionally incredible for your brain and soul. Next time you are looked with an unpleasant circumstance, taking a walk or moving could be a sound outlet for your restless sentiments.

Finally, in the event that you are having an awful day and wind up going after that crate of treats, don't go excessively hard on yourself. Regardless of whether you enjoy emotional eating — wake up and start crisp the following day! Gaining from your encounters and having an uplifting frame of mind can assist you with making an arrangement to dodge these yearnings later on. At the point when you choose to make a move and stop emotional eating remember this is all separated from the voyage. By figuring out how to perceive your conduct and endeavour to transform, you can figure out how to quit being an emotional eater and can, in the long run, accomplish your long-haul objectives.

Chapter 6: The First Principle: Reject the Diet Mentality

At the point when we were a child, your folks presumably set down guidelines about eating, similar to "No treat until you exhaust the baked beans." As a grown-up, you set your very own principles for what to consume and when, and you may choose what great eating intends to you.

In case you're hoping to make your nourishments routine cleaner and more advantageous as long as possible, a couple of straightforward proclamations can assist you with making an arrangement for good eating. Truly, slimming down doesn't work. Instead, it often leaves us preoccupied with food rules and obsessed with maintaining a specific number on the scale.

Ditch the diet for good! Embrace intuitive eating- a flexible style of eating where you primarily follow your internal sensation of hunger and fullness to gauge when, how, and what to eat. Intuitive eating shows respect, trust, and love toward your body. Change your lifestyle and develop an association with nourishment and yourself while following these principles.

Moving Forward

Rejecting the eating routine mindset is an essential yet extremely testing venture. Toss out the eating routine books and magazine articles that offer you bogus any expectation of getting more fit rapidly, effectively, and for all time. Blow up at the falsehoods that have driven you to perceive as though you were a disappointment each time another eating regimen quit working, and you recovered the majority of the weight. In the event that you permit even one little would like to wait that another and better diet may be prowling around the bend, it will keep you from being allowed to revitalize Intuitive Eating. With regards to advancing wellbeing, how we eat is similarly as significant as what we eat; the initial step of natural eating is to make a promise to believe your gut with regards to nourishment decisions.

The initial step of grasping Intuitive Eating is about your way of thinking on nourishment, your body, work out, and so forth. Before we start discussing what Intuitive Eating is, we need to eliminate any confusion air in our brains and reject something called the "diet mentality." Another eating regimen turns out pretty much consistently in the news, each encouraging brisk weight reduction and critical life improvement. It very well may be so enticing to become tied up with the possibility that "this one will be the one that makes a huge difference." And subtly, a significant number of us really need those standards and limitations to give us a guide for what to consume in light of the fact that we haven't the smallest thought.

Diets take numerous structures. They can be the self-evident "official weight control plans" (for example ketogenic, low-carb, Paleo, blood classification, gluten-free, veggie lover, and so on.) yet, in addition, can include:

- Counting calories or carbs/fat/protein

- Counting focuses (Weight Watchers)

- Eating just at specific occasions of the day (irregular fasting or even simply declining to eat past a specific time around evening time)

- Paying compensation for eating "awful" nourishments

- Pacifying hunger by devouring eating routine nourishments

You may have even attempted a quota of these yourself. I'm certain it worked for some time; however, in the end, you surrendered and chose you couldn't do it any longer. You presumably felt like a disappointment, and like you had no restraint. In any case, I'm here to let you know... "You are not the issue. Eating less junk food is the issue". The eating regimen industry knows this and has even begun to change the language they use to bait you in.

Rather than saying the messy word "diet" they are utilizing expressions like "way of life change," "free-form," "mentality," and "clean eating." Toward the day's end, tragically, it's something very similar bundled in an alternate manner.

Why are most individuals on a diet journey? It's a well-known fact. About 95% of people who seek after abstaining from excessive food intake do as such to get in shape. The tragic truth is that abstaining from excessive food intake has not been demonstrated to work for a longer period. Most health food nuts re-put on weight lost inside two years and end up with a large group of reactions including brought down confidence, body disappointment, eased back digestion, and mental damage, including disarranged eating or an all-out dietary problem.

Dismissing the eating regimen attitude (otherwise known as dismissing eating less junk food) is an alarming area. In case you aren't following an eating regimen – what will occur? What will your body do? In what capacity will you eat? There are numerous feelings of dread that can sustain the requirement for a "wellbeing net" of abstaining from excessive food intake and the longing for control around nourishment.

How might we move past these apprehensions and investigate another perspective about nourishment and wellbeing? Here are a few stages to assist you with changing gears and set an establishment for the long haul, economic practices that you can really appreciate.

1. Perceive the worthlessness of consuming fewer calories by investigating your history with eating fewer carbs.

Go through in any event 15 minutes to make a course of events of diets you've been on. Evaluate an amazing amount that has been spent on/off diets. As you make your course of events, ask yourself:

- How much time and cash has been spent?

- Did any eating routine really give you what you needed?

- Any effect on confidence?

- How could you feel about the eating regimen?

- How could you search for nourishment?

- How regularly did nourishment certainties precede delight?

- Any effect on public activity or connections?

Think about how diets have served you (or not served you) and ask yourself, for what reason would I keep on doing likewise again and again, yet anticipate various outcomes? What amount of my life would I like to spend fixating on nourishment and my body? Am I doing this since I love my body or detest my body? Am I progressively significant on the off chance that I occupy less room?

2. Become aware of the diet mentality, thinking, and traits.

Some basic words or expressions that can play in a health food nut's brain are: resolve, dutifulness, fizzling, great, terrible, cheat day, control, blame, disgrace, calories, stuffing, thin, clean, and garbage. High contrast pondering nourishment and exercise resembles attempting to inhale through a straw – you can do it for some time – yet inevitably you need to tear the straw out and take a full breath. This is the dieters' dilemma

Dieting really builds desires and sentiments of being crazy around nourishment. Oftentimes when we are advised not to accomplish something, it can make us feel defiant and denied, which can inevitably prompt yielding. We, at that point, feel remorseful and that we have "no resolve," which can disgrace winding us into negative practices. At the point when we expel the prescriptive guidelines, we would then be able to start to assemble trust in our capacity to self-manage our nourishment admission and settle on decisions that respect our wellbeing and our taste buds.

3. Supplant the scale with self-sympathy.

Probably the greatest device in the eating less junk food world is the scale. It is regularly the driving perspective on "progress." The reality is that the scale doesn't disclose to us anything other than our association with gravity. It doesn't disclose to you how important you are, the way meriting adoration and acknowledgment you are, your body synthesis, or how "solid" you are at the top of the priority list and body. It is essentially a series of digits. In the consuming fewer calories attitude, notwithstanding, this number can make a mess of dramatization and disturb the undertaking to assemble a positive organization with your body and brain.

Instead of weighing in on the scale, look at how you talk to yourself with regards to nourishment and your body. Is there a distinction between how you address yourself versus a dear companion or relative who might be battling? Rehearsing self-sympathy encourages you to manufacture flexibility, acknowledge helplessness, and take on new difficulties. With time, you will find that the additionally minding and steady you are towards yourself, the more probable you will be to change unhelpful practices or thought designs.

Consuming fewer calories isn't the response to carrying on with a solid way of life. It will just prompt frustration, disgrace, and conceit. So how about we abandon that mindset and proceed onward forward into something new! Remember that we live in a culture soaks with ethical quality around bodies and nourishments. Diet culture is for all intents and purposes, a religion that is unpreventable. Be tolerant as you figure out how to relinquish the eating routine mindset and reconnect with your inborn capacity to sustain yourself without dread or confinements.

Chapter 7: The Second principle: Honor your Hunger

The diet mentality has become so entrenched in our culture to the extent that individuals believe the ability to restrict food is just a matter of willpower. But it is more complicated than that. Attempting to remotely control a natural drive as basic as craving can trigger a drive to indulge, and upset the body's finely tuned sign of appetite and saturation. Long periods of overlooking our bodies' prompts and organizing outside nourishment standards can meddle with our capacity to encounter and translate our body's appetite signals. In the event that this is you, it's not your shortcoming. The eating routine culture we live in persuades us we have to control and even overlook our hunger. If you are hungry, that means you need to eat. We are brought into the world instinctive eaters.

Consider babies — they cry when they are eager and stop people in their tracks when they are full. They aren't stressed over bits, calories or craze eat fewer carbs. It is just through our way of life that we are educated generally. Be that as it may, have no dread! You can get back on top of your craving once more. To some people, they cannot remember a time when they were not dieting or following a set of food rules, so they do not even know where to start! What I see regularly is that individuals are panicked; they will constantly eat once they start, or they have lost all craving signals totally.

I have had friends, relatives, individuals, and colleagues all disclose to me that they could go a whole day without eating since they are simply not ravenous. This isn't what we need. An indispensable advance in turning into an instinctive eater is figuring out how to respect your craving. Be that as it may, how is this conceivable when you don't feel hungry? Firstly, let crush the hurdles why we have lost our craving and why we can't generally eat as per our appetite. As such, for what reason would we say we are so disengaged from our bodies? These could act as an aftereffect of the three factors in any case:

- One reason for losing our hunger signals stems from dieting.
- long haul prescription or substance use
- Emotions, for example, tension, apprehension, and living in a steady condition of pressure.

At the point when we have no inward craving prompts, we either don't eat, or we eat as per our own musings and decisions around nourishment (what we or society esteem as "great" or "awful"). By the day's end, this methodology for eating or dealing with our weight doesn't end well. It can cause a fixation around these nourishment rules, which could prompt a dietary issue. We could likewise swing to the far edge of the pendulum and enter the limit – gorge cycle.

I need you to realize that I see that it is so terrifying to lose trust with your body and dread what could occur on the off chance that you let go of control. I guarantee that you can sign a partnership deal with your body. So how would you start re-fabricating that association again and respecting your craving?

Stage One: Eat Enough

A starved body won't furnish you with the exact sign of appetite or totality. This may require searching out a dietary issue treatment community for help, or it might require beginning with eating three suppers and two snacks day by day. When eating less junk food and hardship have been stopped, and you are reliably nourishing your body, you, at that point, should back off and get calm. The way to regarding your craving is to tune in for it.

Stage Two: Perfect Timing

Hunger looks and sounds changed for everybody, so you must turn into a criminologist and distinguish what sensations show up during yearn for you. I urge you to begin tuning in around 1 or 2 hours after dinner or bite. In the event that you are working or feeling on edge, place your hand on your paunch and take two or three full breaths to point out your body. Yearning may start as snarling clamors originating from your stomach, tipsiness, trouble concentrating, peevishness, or migraines. For a few, they may begin having considerations about their next dinner. At 3 or 4 hours after a feast, check-in with yourself. Have a go at asking yourself how hungry you are on a size of 1-10.

Stage Three: Don't Judge

The most significant thing you can do when you notice appetite is to not pass judgment on it. My preferred statement from Intuitive Eating is: "Craving is an ordinary, invited body signal that ought to be grasped. It's an indication that you are getting back in contact with your body's needs." This will result in building greater trust and also will allow you to tune in much easier to the many different signals your body may send. I personally find that the more present I am throughout the day, the better I can take care of myself. Sometimes I notice my vitality is getting low and it's a great opportunity to eat something or different occasions I understood my breath has turned out to be shallow, my heart has started hustling, and I could profit by some full breaths to quiet me down and take me back to the present minute. This enables me to get back in contact with what my body needs.

Step Four: Learn What hunger Feels Like

What does hunger feel like to you? In case you're truly not certain what yearning feels like to you, it's a great opportunity to tune in. When you've gone a timeframe without eating, and you smell or see extremely scrumptious nourishment, how does that make you feel? A few people have wellbeing conditions or are taking prescriptions that may meddle with their yearning signals. It doesn't mean your body is broken. For certain individuals, appetite can inspire Fatigue, grumbly, snarling or burbly, stomach, Stomach pain, Weakness, and Inability to concentrate.

This brings back the memory of having this conversation with a colleague of mine when I was in my 20s, and I explained my stomach had a painful burning sensation when I was hungry. He was determined that yearning didn't feel along these lines and that I was causing it to up. Try not to give individuals a chance to discredit your sentiments. You are the master of your own body.

Step Five: Understand Your Hunger/Fullness Scale

I will believe I am crystal clear. I said "YOUR" not "THE" in light of the fact that everybody encounters craving and completion in various manners. Basically, a craving/totality scale is a scale at which the least end is your most eager, and the best quality is your generally full. Commonly this is viewed as a 1 to 10 where 1 is the point at which you have an inclination that you're starving to death, and 10 is the point at which you are so stuffed that you're on the verge of sickness.

You start to comprehend what your body is letting you know, and thus, you respect that by bolstering your body what it needs when it needs. It additionally averts that fixation on nourishment that happens when you get excessively ravenous.

Step Six: Feed Your Body What it is Hungry For

As mentioned earlier, when you listen to your body's hunger cues and feed it accordingly, you build body trust. There are many ways to facilitate this process. Here are some ideas:

- Keep delicious, supporting bites close by consistently

- Meal plan and prep

- Stash simple dinners in the cooler

- Stock your home with an assortment of fun nourishments

Some individuals don't accept they ought to eat, in any event, when they are eager. Or then again a few people recognize what they are eager for (instance: a treat) however eat another nourishment (for instance: a rice cake. Then again. This isn't honoring your body's hunger. Another scenario is on poolside party Carole where Liya and her friends sit at a table laden with gorgeous nuts, fruits, and pastries. "it's okay, my diet begins after eating cake," says Liya, excusing herself as she reaches for another slice of cake that what her body metabolism could conceive at that time which spurs her friends to laugh in agreement, and the ladies were all in agreement to swear off cake after the party.

In all, while most diets expect you to oppose a snarling stomach, natural eating is tied in with modifying confidence in your body's signals. You'll figure out how to be increasingly mindful of your craving and how to react properly to it before you become insatiable. Attempt this at home: Before every supper, rate your degree of craving, write down a couple of inward prompts that you watched, and the hour of the day. Do this for a week, and you'll turn out to be more on top of your hunger, just as which nourishments convey enduring vitality and those that are quick consuming.

Chapter 8: The Third Principle – Be Content with Nourishment

Our lifestyle has done an amazingly unbelievable work of making us believe a couple of sustenance are "awful," and others are "extraordinary." At the point when we hear this kind of verbiage, it convinces there are nourishment sources we should and should not eat. So, we make a once-over of guidelines for ourselves... I'll eat this one; I won't eat this one, etc. Instinctive eating advances that nourishment ought to consistently be a real existence improving knowledge. Exactly when you preclude sustenance, you will have the alternative to avoid it from the outset. You'll probably feel incredibly happy for your self-restraint. Regardless, as time goes on, your opinions of hardship increase, and the sustenance end up being continuously engaging. Sooner or later, you land at a tipping point. You eat the sustenance. However, since you bound for so long, you will end up eating significantly more than you regularly would, inciting extraordinary fault and disfavor.

Note: Nourishment should not make you feel deficiency and lack of regard.

We empower sustenance to make us feel these things since we are giving it a power it was never planned to have in our lives. What you eat doesn't portray who you are as a person. You are "terrible" for eating broccoli or "horrendous" for eating brownies. You are made in the picture of God, and that makes you typically significant.

I review it being such assistance to finally relinquish the conviction that my value relied upon the sustenance I ate. I comprehended the measure of my real character I could look for after once I released this obsession and made amicability with sustenance. I have a lot of inclusion with confining nourishment along these lines, making me need it much more. One nourishment that I, in every case, truly battled with, was nutty spread. At the point when I was eating fewer carbs, I used to turn out to be so baffled at how rapidly my everyday assignment of nourishment would diminish when I consolidated nutty spread. Regardless I had it; however, there were ordinarily I enjoyed in light of the fact that I had subliminally made a shortage encompassing it.

I went the extent that creation my significant other shrouds the nutty spread in our home (on various occasions really) on the grounds that once I began having it, I couldn't quit eating it. I thought I was by and large "great" by having him conceal it or not in any event, getting it at the store. The way toward causing harmony with nourishment can require some investment relying upon what number of nourishments you have had on your "prohibited rundown."

They prescribe taking each nourishment in turn and making harmony with it. So how might you do it? It's fundamental - give yourself unequivocal approval to eat. Genuinely, I am a sustenance master, and really, I just said you can give yourself the approval to eat whatever, at whatever point. This movement is one of the most noteworthy walks in transforming into an instinctual eater since it retrains your brain to begin pondering sustenance in a morally fair manner and to trust in your body truly. This looks like the accompanying: Disposing of your musings of explicit sustenance being "dreadful" and "incredible."

Nourishment can't avoid being sustenance! Dietary advantage may fluctuate between sustenance, yet at this stage, we're not worried over that. Your mental wellbeing and relationship with sustenance are needed. Eating what you really need. Make an effort not to condemn your desires. Your body will need what it needs. From the outset, you should work through desires that started from whole deal hardship; however, as time goes on, those will leave.

Longings are your partner! Eating without making up for it. Contradict the drive to rehearse more, limit more, or somehow compensate for something you ate. You don't need to win the benefit to eat - you reserve the option to eat basically because you are alive! So now, I appreciate what you're thinking… this startling!

Envision a situation wherein I don't stop eating. Think about how conceivable it is that I simply eat solidified yogurt for an astonishing leftover portion.

Think about how conceivable it is that I can't trust myself. In any case, here's the improving truth - when you understand you can really have anything you want, the exceptional needs to eat will diminish. Likewise, the more you open yourself to that sustenance you're so terrified of, the less you will pine for them. (Studies show this thought - it's called habituation, and it's genuinely cool). Likewise, to the degree sustenance goes, we'll get to that later - for the present, take care of business it to express that refreshingly, your body is your partner. It's the perfect open door for the sustenance fight to end. What I understand now in the wake of becoming familiar with instinctive eating is that I had really made it illegal nourishment.

In this manner, I made nourishment that I needed in overabundance just on the grounds that I didn't give myself unlimited authorization to have it. Need to realize how enticing nutty spread is to me since I have grasped instinctive eating? Not in any manner. A few days, I have it. A few days, I don't. Be that as it may, I never gorge on it any longer or feel on edge about the amount I have had, on the grounds that I realize I can have anyway a lot of I need. I have discovered that spoonful after spoonful just makes me feel horrible. Presently, I put some on a cut of bread, and that is sufficient for me. It leaves me fulfilled, and unexpectedly, I don't as a rule need anything else than that. Envision my amazement following quite a while of this nourishment having command over me.

The way toward causing harmony with nourishment can require some investment relying upon what number of food sources you have had on your "prohibited rundown." They suggest taking each nourishment in turn and making harmony with it. Likewise, here is different techniques or standards to discover a feeling of happiness with nourishment. The accompanying advances are the immediate standards and the means you can take towards harmony with nourishment and your body: Focus on the nourishments that are speaking to you and make a rundown of them. Put a check by the nourishments you really eat, at that point, circle remaining nourishments that you've been limiting. Give yourself the authorization to eat one prohibited nourishment from your rundown, by then go to the store and purchase this nourishment, or request it at a café.

Check-in with yourself to check whether the nourishment tastes comparable to you envisioned. In case you find that you truly like it, keep on giving yourself the authorization to purchase or request it. Ensure that you keep enough of the nourishment in your kitchen, so you realize that it will be there in case you need it. Or then again, if that appears to be excessively unnerving, go to an eatery and request the specific nourishment as frequently as you like. When you make harmony with one nourishment, proceed with your rundown until all of the nourishments are attempted, assessed, and liberated. This procedure will remove the longing from the nourishments you have been confining.

The initial couple of times you do it, you may enjoy or gorge on them… you are not a disappointment that you do this. In any case, keep on enabling yourself to have it, I figure what you will discover is that specific nourishment will lose its control over you. Sooner or later, our bodies state, 'No more.' At the start of Intuitive Eating, numerous individuals surrender since they are feeling like they are eating excessively… this inclination passes. It might take weeks, or a while, however, it should pass in the event that you are truly tuning in to your craving and totality signals. To wind up fruitful at natural eating, you should likewise move toward becoming receptive to your body's satiety signs.

You can confide in yourself to turn into an Intuitive Eater. When you strip away the layers of diet culture and principles, your body genuinely comprehends what it needs. It might require some investment to arrive; however, you can completely recover trust with your body and with nourishment. Your body is so keen, and it can let you know precisely what it needs in case you enable it to. What is the contrast between Intuitive Eating and Mindful Eating? I utilized the terms Mindful Eating and Intuitive Eating reciprocally. While this isn't absolutely off base, it's critical to take note of the distinctions.

The Center for Mindful Eating characterizes careful eating as "enabling yourself to wind up mindful of the positive and supporting open doors that are accessible through nourishment choice and readiness by regarding your own internal knowledge" and "utilizing using all of your resources faculties in eating nourishment that is both fulfilling to you and sustaining to your body and getting to be mindful of physical craving and satiety prompts to control your choices to start and end eating." You can tell in that spot that Intuitive Eating includes the standards of careful eating.

Anyway, it goes above and beyond, additionally tending to the significance of dismissing the abstaining from excessive food intake attitude regarding your body (paying little heed to your weight or shape), adapting to passionate eating, and delicate development and sustenance without judgment. Both careful eating and Intuitive Eating can be valuable apparatuses to help you with arriving at a position of typical eating.

Chapter 9: The Fourth Principle – Challenging the Food Police.

The Food Police are the musings in your mind that pronounce you as "great" for having a plate of mixed greens for lunch and "terrible" on the grounds that you ate dessert/carbs/sugar/and so forth. These are the irrational decides that were made by eating fewer carbs that reason you to feel remorseful. These guidelines are housed somewhere down in your cerebrum and spring up every day to administer your nourishment choices. It is difficult to view eating like a typical, pleasurable movement when the nourishment police have tight. Testing the nourishment police is a significant advance towards turning into an instinctive eater.

The Food Police is the profoundly inserted musings, sentiments, feelings that we have received through the span of numerous years from different weight control plans, articles, companions, family, specialists, and so on. The Food Police is that thought in our mind that is revealing to us what is "great" or "terrible" and screens every one of the "rules" we have made for ourselves dependent on our past encounters with how we have nourished our body.

At the point when I began to make look into, I thought it would have been pretty much every one of the individuals' assessments I hear consistently, whether it is face to face or in my web-based life feed. While that is a piece of the Food Police, really, the greater piece of the condition is in our very own heads and the guidelines we have chosen to pursue dependent on our past encounters with abstinent from enormous food intake. I have been on numerous eating regimens since I started my slimming down voyage, and I have heard a ton of standards throughout the years.

In the Intuitive Eating book, they depict the Food Police as a "solid voice that is created through counting calories. It is your inward judge and jury that decides whether you are doing "great" or "terrible." It is the total of all your eating fewer carbs and nourishment administers, and gets more grounded with each diet. It likewise gets fortified through new nourishment decides that you may find out about in magazines or messages you get notification from companions or family".

Coming up next are a portion of the couple of things my Food Police say to me;

- I ought not to eat an excess of bread.

- I ought not to let my children eat an excess of sugar.

- I feel like a terrible Mom on the off chance that I give my children juice.

- I ought not to be ravenous yet; I didn't eat that sometime in the past.

- I ought not to drink espresso the half and half is so terrible for me so

- I ought to figure out how to like it dark.

- You didn't get enough advances today.

- Even if you are pregnant, it doesn't mean you should "let yourself go."

We, as a whole, have those inward voices that shout at us once in a while. A few days, the voices can be quieted, and different days; it requires a great deal of exertion and profound breathing, to quiet it down!

How am I testing the Food Police?

Ordinary, I remind myself why I have picked Intuitive Eating. I help myself to remember the model I am setting and how the decisions I am making have a far-reaching influence on the lives of my kids and their bliss with their own bodies. Bodies that are solid and solid and have a solid instinct at this moment. The more they can eat instinctively before they hear messages in school and media, the better. I rather not be the individual who starts to disclose to them that being dainty methods, you are better or that specific nourishments are "awful."

The majority of us were destined to eat naturally, except if there was neediness, ailing health, bolstering tubes, and so forth included, at that point, those kids should figure out how to discover their instinct with respect to appetite and totality. My objective is a solid establishment of body acknowledgment for my youngsters.

What's more, they have to uncover that from me. Acknowledgment isn't tolerating a pal that is flimsy or fit since that is the thing that the general public let us know. Acknowledgment is realizing we are powering our bodies such that we feel our best, we move our bodies since it makes them feel better and we practice self-consideration since that makes us more joyful as a whole, they not are attached to the number on the scale or the manner in which our body looks.

The Food Police Keeps Nourishment and Our Body at War.

I don't think about you, yet the battling gets old sooner or later. The consistent spotlight on what was on my plate and how that was going to impact my weight got depleting. II need to be sound and feel better; however, that is more than being dainty.

It is additionally not being excessively devoured by nourishment or exercise and how my body will react to them. I needed to figure out how to believe that on the off chance that I figure out how to tune in to my body, it will deal with me. As my adventure proceeds in Intuitive Eating, I am fortifying different voices that would talk about on this part:

The Food Anthropologist

This voice enables me to find new nourishments without passing judgment on ourselves. It enables me to respect the musings and sentiments I am having about how my body is being encouraged without making a decision about them dependent on what another person figures I ought to eat or do. Nobody else can disclose to you what your body needs. We, as a whole, need various things, and what makes one individual feel great doesn't mean it will make everybody feel better. All things considered, you additionally need to arrive at a point that you can "hear" what your body is letting you know. Acknowledgment is realizing we are filling our bodies such that we feel our best, we move our bodies since it makes them feel better and we practice self-consideration since that makes us more joyful as such, they are not attached to the number on the scale or the manner in which our body looks.

The Nurturer-this voice is delicate and is the means by which we would converse with our closest companions or close relatives. This voice is the means by which we converse with a companion who is battling with decisions they have made. Here are a few models; "You are not terrible that you had one treat" "It is alright that you avoided your exercise since you were worn out.

Rest is similarly as significant as development" "You are still YOU, regardless of what the scale says" "At the point when you deal with yourself you are more joyful" This voice isn't an "excuser", it is really a voice of reason and self-consideration and what I have discovered is self-consideration is so significant when learning instinctive eating. At the point when we become an Intuitive Eater, we realize what we like and what we are doing.

On the off chance that you are understanding this and think you just like desserts and sweet and seared nourishment. I am here to disclose to you I would profoundly question it. Your body will start to hunger for sustenance, and when you figure out how to hear it out after some time, the yearnings for the nourishments you have doubtlessly confined for such a long time die down.

That doesn't mean you never eat them or don't need them; you simply acknowledge how your body feels when having them in contrast with different things, and you figure out how to give yourself what makes your body feel it is ideal. At the point when I went to dietary issue treatment ten years back, my Food Police had an extremely strong grip on me. I had SO MANY RULES. Throughout the years, I have gradually discharged a few. At the point when I quit eating fewer carbs not long ago, I have focused on discharging the guidelines I was not in any case mindful I had put on myself. It is a procedure. It doesn't happen without any anticipation, and harmony isn't constantly found rapidly. Be that as it may, it is conceivable.

I have consumed a greater part of my time on earth on an eating regimen or attempting to change the manner in which my body searches for one reason or the other. Closing down the desires and principles, I have set for myself is a procedure I have focused on, regardless of to what extent it takes. A few days are superior to other people, a few days, I end up making statements that are hurtful; however, the distinction in me today and the individual I was a year back is I perceive the mischief now. My best isn't an impression of the scale; it is an appearance by the way I am feeling.

Chapter 10: The Fifth Principles: Respect Your Fullness

Respecting your fullness means listening for the signals your body sends when it's satisfied, approaching fullness, and full — and making choices about whether to stop or continue eating, considering what your body is telling you. In a nutshell, respecting your fullness means not eating past fullness.

Respecting your fullness will help you arrive at the weight where your body is happiest and healthiest. This is also the weight that will be easiest for you to maintain long term. Keep in mind – losing and recapturing weight is more destructive to your body and mind than remaining at a heavier weight. Honoring your craving and regarding your totality are various sides of a similar coin. The two of them include careful eating and body trust. Despite your past or current dietary patterns, you can regard your totality. It takes some training; however, you can arrive. An expert can help, particularly in the event that you end up habitually indulging or suspect you may have voraciously consuming food issues.

Sometimes you listen to the body flag that discloses to you that you are never again eager. Watch the signs that show that you're easily full. Respite in a dinner or nourishment and ask yourself how the nourishment tastes, and what is your present completion level? Perhaps a few steps with analogy would be sufficient to juxtapose.

Step one: Tune in While You Eat

So many of us eat meals while watching television, watching a video on our phones, scrolling through social media, or while on our emails. Consider it — when's the last time you taken a seat at a table and did nothing other than eating (and maybe chat with your feasting accomplice)?

To be completely honest: I here and there eat before screens. What's more, I additionally try sitting at my eating table with no screens (or even webcasts) and making the most of my supper.

My accomplice works late a ton, so frequently, I'm doing this without anyone else. Instead of thinking about this as a desolate encounter, I'm appreciative I have the way to set up a dinner and altogether appreciate it. So, what does it resemble to be careful while eating? Preferably you'd tune in with your yearning before you start eating.

You could consider where you are on the appetite/totality scale. At that point, you'd start eating, biting each chomp altogether, and relishing the flavor, fragrance, and surface of your nourishment. You will set down your utensils every so often, maybe take a taste of water. You'll take a gander at your nourishment.

What's more, the part route through eating, you'll tune in with your body and think about where you are on the yearning/totality scale. Is it true that you are as yet eager? It is safe to tell that you are getting full? In a perfect world, we'd push away our plates at around a 7 out of 10 on the scale. This implies you're easily full, however, not overstuffed. You're not awkward, and you're never again eager or pondering or inspired by nourishment. You're fulfilled.

Stage Two: Stop When You're Full

What does completion feel like to you? Nonattendance of appetite, an extended stomach, never again keen on nourishment are large signs that you're getting full. The important thing is to stop when you're feeling enjoyably full and before you feel awkwardly full.

You realize you're full; however, you need to continue eating. Presently what? Wonder why that might be. Is it nourishment you don't typically enable yourself to have? The significant reason for indulging is a limitation. Consider it: in the event that you realize you can have any nourishment whenever you need, what might drive you to indulge it?

Let assume there is specific nourishment you avoid in light of the fact that you think you'll pig out yourself on it, it's an ideal opportunity to open up access to that nourishment. It may appear to be unreasonable, yet it's much the same as telling a child they can't have or accomplish something — at that point, that is all they need! At the point when you're full yet at the same time have delightful nourishment on your plate, spare that nourishment for later, and remind yourself you can have it at whatever point you need. You are regarding your totality.

You're avoiding that feeling of distress. You're doing what is best for your body at this moment.

What's more, you can eat at whatever point you need! Consider the possibility that you're hesitant to eat to the point of completion. This is regular in individuals who have scattered eating. In any case, experiencing life constantly hungry is an unacceptable quality of life. Peevishness, mind haze, low vitality, and nourishment distraction are unpleasant. It's important to nourish yourself until you're full to build that give-and-take body trust.

Practice reinforcing your inner knowing of fullness and that the bite in your mouth is your last. Nudge your plate forward, put your utensils or napkin in your plate, wrap up the food as leftovers - do what you need to do to stand by your decision. Remember, you can and will eat again. You are finished with this snack or meal.

Remember, by honoring your hunger in the very beginning; it is much easier to recognize your fullness. You have to confide in your body to disclose to you when what, and the amount to eat and your body will confide in you to bolster it when what and the amount it needs.

Step Three: Accept That Overeating Happens

Holidays, Vacations, Emotional times, Nourishment frailty, Insane calendars, and Drugs. There are numerous reasons we gorge, and that is absolutely typical. Keep in mind that instinctive eating isn't a yearning/totality diet. At times we eat, and some of the time, we gorge. It's an unavoidable truth. It's likewise typical to indulge nourishment on the off chance that you've quite recently given yourself unrestricted consent to eat it.

It's a normal piece of the nourishment opportunity process. Realize that things will adjust in time. In the event that you wind up feeling wild with nourishment and reliably eating exceptionally a lot of nourishment as well as to an entirely awkward express, it's a great opportunity to see an expert.

You can be as readied and careful as physically conceivable and still wind up in circumstances where you're eating close to nothing or to an extreme. Give yourself a little room to breathe. The crucial thing to recollect is there will never be a need to confine in the wake of gorging. This equitable sustains that hurtful eating regimen/gorge cycle. Make sure to confide in your body to disclose to you what it needs. You may get yourself normally less eager following a day of indulging. Or then again not. There is no set-in-stone.

Stage Four: Give Yourself Unconditional Permission to Eat

Respecting your fullness means you can acknowledge when your body has had enormous to eat biologically, and this principle relies heavily on unequivocal authorization to eat (Principle 3: Make Peace with Food).

How can you leave food inside the bowl if you are unsure when you'll be able to eat that food or meal again? Respecting your fullness, stopping eating when you are full, becomes simpler when you know you'll be able to eat food again when you become hungry.

Step Five: Engage in Sense Perception and Really Taste the Food.

Ask yourself how your food tastes. How does it smell? Notice the mouthfeel, the temperature, its palatability. Is it worthy of your taste buds, or are you simply eating because the food is in front of you? Remember, just as we can give ourselves permission to eat the foods we do like, it's okay to say "no, thank you!" to the ones we do not like or want at that moment. You are in charge of what and the amount you eat. However, when figuring out how to regard your completion and quit eating when fulfilled, recollect the following apart from the step I provided above trust two there love in partnership if you could find one. Combining the steps and this axiom together will help you the target audience of fullness.

Dispensing with interruptions can truly assist you with tuning into your body's endeavors to impart when it is fulfilled, full, or still eager. If you are perusing, talking, sitting in front of the television, perusing the web, or wandering off in fantasy land, it will be barely noticeable your body's endeavors to reveal to you it has had enough. Eat gradually. It requires some investment for your body to register that it is satisfied.

Eating slowly will help make sure that you don't get too full before your body has had the time to register that it's had enough. If you are really enjoying a portion of food and want to continue eating for the taste, even though you recognize your hungry free, remember you can finish it later. Put it aside and check back with yourself an hour later to see if you are hungry again. If so, eat some more. If not, wait until you are hungry.

You will enjoy the food even more if you eat it when you are hungry! Have faith in your body to disclose to you when to stop and when to keep eating – you CAN leave it inside your bowl and return back for more. Your mind may try and take over and make rules and restrictions (or justify eating when you're already satisfied), but only your body knows what it needs in any situation.

Dieting has allowed your mind to be in charge for years. It's time to let the true expert – your body- take charge. Respecting your fullness requires that you also respect your hunger. It is difficult to eat slowly and mindfully when you have to let yourself get too hungry. Try not to give all the emphasis on the sign of totality a chance to shield you from making the most of your nourishment.

Chapter 11: The Sixth Principle: Discover the Satisfaction Factor

It's important to remember that food is not just fuel. Food is a form of self-care, and it should be enjoyable. You deserve to treat yourself, and hat refers to what, how, and where you're eating. That is an extraordinary ability to have; however, we likewise should recollect that totality and fulfilment are not really something very similar. You can be physically full yet not be fulfilled for an assortment of reasons you didn't eat what you were needing; your supper was feeling the loss of a key segment (carbs, fat, or protein), and so on.

The fulfilment factor is one of the most dominant controllers of our eating. Incidentally, it is the primary concern we pass up when we confine/diet! Maslow discloses to us that we are driven by neglected needs. At the point when we deny ourselves what we need, we wind up eating more and getting a charge out of less — battling against our bodies as opposed to confiding in them. This is one of the principal reasons the eating routine mindset simply doesn't work.

At the point when we eat what we genuinely need and we eat enough to be full, we begin to accept we can confide in our bodies to lead us to the correct nourishments and the perfect sums. As this trust develops, we start to find that our bodies work admirably of automatic both the sum and sort of nourishment we hunger for. We don't have to totally wipe out nutrition classes or make different standards. Our bodies do what needs to be done for us… and we likewise get the additional advantage of really getting a charge out of the things we eat. Envision that! That aside, let be completely clear at this point. When you consider nourishment, how frequently does your own fulfilment become possibly the most important factor?

Do you:

- Ask yourself what may taste great? Have you at any point heard somebody state they have a sweet tooth? Or on the other hand, possibly you've heard somebody state they favor salty bites? Do you know what your flavor inclination will, in general, be? Presently it is a decent time to explore and set aside some effort to think about your faculties. Do you like nourishments that are flavorful, sweet, severe, tart, rich, salty, hot, somewhat smoky, or tasteless? What surfaces do you like? Do you like crunchy, chewy, or velvety? Do your inclinations change consistently and with the seasons? Does the manner in which your nourishment is plated have any kind of effect on you? Utilize your faculties! Attempt various nourishments and carry attention to whether that nourishment is something you would need to eat once more. Or on the other hand,

- do you, in general, set aside the nourishments you most appreciate for 'more beneficial' options?

Think about a period you went out to eat at an eatery. You may have been looking at a cheeseburger on the menu; however, at that point, out of blame, requested a serving of mixed greens. Be that as it may, it's an ideal opportunity to ask yourself what you really need to eat, not what you ought to eat. Think about which nourishments taste great to you, and you anticipate eating. Here and there, you have confined ourselves to nourishments for such a long time that you experience difficulty making sense of what it is that you like.

Did you know?

Fulfilment is extremely the centre point of Intuitive Eating. Every one of the rest of the standards 9 of Intuitive Eating joins some component of fulfillment, regardless of whether it is with your body, your brain, or your taste buds. Human is intended to get delighted and fulfillment from our suppers. The nonappearance of that fulfilment factor regularly needs you wanting for additional, however, recall Rome was not worked in a day. Here are a few stages to assist you with recovering fulfilment in eating...

Stage One: Ask Yourself What You Really Want to Eat.

Instead of attempting to have the 'sound' adaptation of what you're desiring (which once in a while hits the spot), have a go at having what you really need. You'll see it much all the more fulfilling. At the point when you reliably enable yourself to do this, you will be considerably more ready to eat a sum that feels better, as opposed to feeling constrained to eat a huge sum since you have denied yourself. In the event that you've lived with nourishment rules for quite a while, you may not really recognize what you like to eat any longer! Set aside the effort to rediscover your one of a kind inclinations. Be happy to attempt new things. No nourishments are forbidden!

Have you, at any point, been eager, state around 3 pm? What you truly need is your preferred chocolate chip treat; however, you have perused that you ought to have an apple. Despite the fact that the apple doesn't sound too great at the present time, you obediently eat it since it's what you 'ought to do.' But, regardless, you feel ravenous and unsatisfied! What's more, presently, your yearnings for that treat are significantly more grounded!

Maybe you attempt to get a yoghurt since that is additionally 'solid' nourishment. You do like yoghurt; however, it's not so much engaging at the present time. In any case, you eat it in any case. Regardless you don't feel right, and afterward, you wind up eating the treat. In any case, rather than getting a charge out of that delectable treat and enjoying it, you're feeling so regretful on the grounds that you were 'frail' and surrendered' to eating the treat.

Consider the possibility that you had recently eaten that treat in any case. How would you imagine that would have changed your experience? So that why it very crucial to know what you really want to because the opportunity cost is not something worthwhile in the long run. The next steps should help bring some more clarity

Step Two: Discover the Pleasure of The Palate.

Taste, texture, aroma, appearance, temperature, and filling-capacity are all components of food that we can experience and enjoy. Can you relate? Perhaps, like me, I always have someone to showcase at every event. Who is mine to blame, that nature for you? I just thought it would be great that I share it. Johnny boy, that the name we called him while in our 20s. His soccer practice schedule had him sitting in my car, in the dark, three nights a week. He would regularly eat these crunchy burger embedded with some creamy vanilla flavor. I can't even picture how or what to call it. For brevity sake, let burger toasters during his hour practice. Not satisfying, right? But here is the brilliant part. That simple act of discovery his palate helped him feel more connected to and satisfied by his food.

Step Three: Make Your Eating Experience More Enjoyable.

Sitting down for a meal with a family member/friend will be much better than standing in front of the fridge...trust me. It could also erupt from how your environment looks like. What is your eating environment like, and does that affect your satisfactory experience when eating?

Here are a couple of proposals to make your condition increasingly wonderful:

- Clear the table. Eating with a pile of papers and books around you sends a not really inconspicuous message that you're not justified, despite any potential benefits.

- Add something to expand the visual intrigue. Maybe a few blooms or the glinting light from a flame.

- Try inconspicuous scents: Some individuals discover the smell of citrus or cinnamon, through blend or a flame, to bring added satisfaction to their eating background.

- Don't overlook sounds: Some instrumental music like jazz or traditional can truly help set the stage. While instrumental music can truly elevate your faculties and help increment your fulfilment with suppers, gadgets like TV, mobile phones, tablets, and books all occupy you from your dinner. I prescribe taking a shot at eating without those present.

Different societies make a staggering showing of making encounters around nourishments. Some European nations go through hours of eating together. At the point when I contemplated abroad in China and Taiwan, I adored the family-style eating. It enabled me to attempt a smidgen of everything and choose what dishes tasted great to me.

Step Four: Check-in Throughout the Meal to See If the Food Still Tastes Good.

This might mean trying a few bites first and seeing what you might want to add in. When I tracked macros, I always thought sauces were a 'waste of calories,' which meant that my food was often dry and relatively tasteless. Make your food nice to eat, and it will be a lot more enjoyable.

The more chomps you take, the less engaging it will taste as you approach satiety. You will appreciate nourishment more on the off chance that you tune in to your appetite and totality prompts! Might find that it takes less nourishment to make you feel fulfilled as you find what food sources taste great and feel better. You likewise may discover on certain days that it takes more nourishment for no clear reason. Both of these are alright! Be nonjudgmental as you manufacture trust with your body, and accept that you were made to be happy with what you eat. At whatever point I request a domino's pizza, in case I'm eating carefully, I will see that the main couple of chomps taste the best. After I'm mostly through, it will, in general, lose its allure. Do you see this with specific nourishments that you eat? I suppose your reply should tend toward the "YES" except for those who are medically unfit or taste deficient.

As you sife through the activities for the sixth principle, remember to enjoy yourself! Making peace with food is not necessarily taking it too serious. Go out of your comfort zone and try new foods, or prepare old recipes from your childhood. Take time to explore the meals that bring you joy.

Chapter 12: The Seventh Principle: Honor Your Feeling Without Using Food

This principle, to many, is the most important of all the principles because it addresses the main problem of excessive food consumption. Many people have taken food as a tool to cover up their emotions and problems. The implication of this is that the problems do not go away, so they continue eating, and invariably abuse food intake. Some people, then again, think that it's hard to stop some specific type of food which in time becomes very bad for their health. When making peace or honoring ones feeling, there should be an understanding that without this procedure or principal, the other principles are nothing but waste.

There are several feelings, for example, outrage, disdain, fear, and several others. The first thing we ought to realize is that until we honor our feelings, we cannot have freedom. The mind is always searching for happiness and peace and sometimes don't care if it is short-termed or long-termed, due to this, eating is sometimes its own way of finding short term happiness, and this needs to stop. It is very important for us to know that the mind of a person loves to fight for what it wants, and because of these, there might be a little problem or restriction from the mind when you start observing this principle. There are things we need to know about honoring our feelings, and they are very important in our wish to progress.

1. **Recognize the problem and its source:**

This is one of the first real ones must face in order to carry out intuitive eating. The problem must first be recognized. There are many people with issues and thoughts but do not know that those thoughts are the cause of their taking in of excess food. Therefore, when an individual acknowledges there is a problem, such a person has begun the first step of making peace with himself and his mind without food. Although this is a huge breakthrough, yet it is not enough to know the problem, you must also know the root of the problem. Some people have an emotional breakdown because of the breakup; it is not enough for such a person to realize it is as a result of the breakup, rather you must also be ready to check the foundation of this problem. It might be your dressing, look, size, language, work, and several other things. Until you discover this, you might not fully recover.

I will be frank to say that recognizing the problem might not be as easy as it sounds in some cases. There are people that can't place their hands on why they eat abnormally. This is because they have been doing this for years and might not be able to place where the reason comes from, perhaps it began with the parent or guardian, either way, such issues can still be addressed if such a person visits a professional.

1. **Be True to Your Feelings:**

This is a very important part of healing; you must be true to your feelings. Accept who you are; many people that hide their emotions by eating have great difficulty getting up from it. There are numerous individuals that conflict with the truth about their feelings. Many patients with anger and patience issues most times want people to believe they are the opposite of what they are. Many times they deceive even themselves that they do not have issues, thereby using food as a means of escape.

1. **Be Determined and Take Actions:**

Although this might sound multinational, it is not enough to recognize a problem, and it's the source, the determination to fight the problem is equally important. The determination to fight the problem should be in us even when we sleep. Taking a person who needs to fight anger, for example, although you have realized the problem and the source, the next thing expected is to have the determination not to be angry for any reason. Therefore, if a reason to get angry comes, the brain will remind us of this determination. Many people are bored; they live their day in boredom and because of these, they eat to take it off.

After discovering the source of this problem, one must be determined to do other things that will help fight boredom, like visiting friends, playing video games, and several others. There are a few people that eat to find forgiveness. Although this situation is not common, it does exist. It is necessary to know that actions differ from problem to problem and people to people.

Some people's issues might only need a strong conviction from within, but others might need group therapy, meditation, yoga; in fact, some might need to see a psychologist. The most significant thing to note about talking about, although it sounds like all you need these just the beginning it cannot solve all your problems. Always doing something productive also helps a lot. You can try traveling, sports, fishing, and several other things.

1. **Ask Yourself Questions**

Many times you will feel the urge to eat more or eat those meals you ought not to eat make it a duty to ask yourself questions like

1) Do I need this?

2) What should I be doing now?

3) By eating this, am I doing myself harm or good?

4) After taking this, will this feeling last?

These questions will not only help you keep watch, but they will likewise assist you with understanding the implication of what you are doing.

1. **Read Positive Books and Stay Around Position Minded People:**

There are many books that can help many types of issues. Reading such books helps the mind at healing. The people with which you stay determine the kind of person you are or will become. Honoring your feelings deals with acceptance. Accepting who you are and not using food as a means of escape. Many group therapies help many people in accepting who they are. Human by nature is a social being, and we crave for acceptance and love, we crave for people who would love us and accept us for who we are. Group therapies not only do these, they also create an avenue of trust. These well for those bothered with secrets and a way out of it.

Although not everyone loves reading, therefore movies or Songs can be an answer to the people that fall under this category regarding people and places. On many occasions, religion has been a huge help to some. The preaching of forgiveness and love that religion preaches have helped a whole lot of people to get better, bury their past, and honor their emotions.

1. **Know It's A Gradual Process**

I know the wish of many to grow out of their habits and distress, however hard you try I am sorry to disappoint you, honoring your mind is a gradual process. Sometimes you will feel down and go back to your habit. However, that should not way you down. Stand up and start over from where you stopped. One thing many people fail to understand that bad diet, wrong diet, and excessive intake of food can sometimes cause an addiction. It is then important for anyone that wants to be free to know that like all addiction issues, it takes time for the healing process to fully occur.

1. **Let Your Story Go:**

Stories are part of us, and we believe our stories are ours, and they belong totally to us. You are not wrong in any way if you think this. However, the story that led you to see food as a way out of your problems has to be thrown away. Although you have accepted who you are and sought help, regardless, you have to throughout that story you are holding on to so as to prepare your mind for a new, beautiful, and better one. The problem with many people is that they do not realize that those stories ought to be left alone. An example of such a story is a rape story. The victim has to realize the horrible story has to be forgotten so that a better story can replace it.

After you have done all of these, you will discover a new form of happiness that does not get triggered by eating rather from yourself. Not just this, you will understand your environment better and have a sense of will. The rate of progress in all you do will be high, and you would have healed to a very large extent from all your traumatic experiences. The seventh principle is not just about intuitive eating; it deals with several aspects of life, and due to these, many people have regarded it as a very important if not the most important of all the principles of principle eating.

Chapter 13: The Eighth Principle: Respect Your Body.

Our distinctiveness is the thing that makes us distinctive in a delightful manner, and our beautiful differences are the thing that makes us unique as individuals. Every individual eve identical twin yet don't have similar fingerprints. Intuitive eating is not an escape from healthy eating or an excuse to junk-eating; rather, it is a way of promoting nature's master plan in our bodies. It is no news that respect is reciprocal while upholding this saying even our bodies are not left out. If you respect your body, it helps you a lot in accepting and celebrating your individuality.

Respecting your body cannot be achieved by just 'wishing' but by knowing yourself and your history. For a lady who happens to come from a family of about 80 percent individuals being on the plus-size range, it is only normal and logical that she comes to the reality of her genetic makeup and enjoy who she is, with this level of understanding, she will not be really bothered about having fried chips with soda drinks on outings or even on causal food breaks. However, understanding your body also requires that you understand foods that make you add flesh without even asking for your permission; thus, saving you from any form of a panic attack such metabolic process may bring on your psychology. It is important to reiterate that intuitive eating wasn't philosophy was not postulated to promote unhealthy eating habits but rather a way of eating properly without the man-made body standards.

In our world today, where body-shaming is not a new word, especially on social media, and even within gossips and chit-chats, people tend to fall under that peer pressure situation, interesting this type of peer pressure is not only found amongst teenagers alone but cuts across all age groups. In other to overcome this particular type of vice, it is important to follow this principle of intuitive eating. "Respect your body" in other words, accept who you are physical. In some part of the world where chubby females have the majority of male suitors and of course, admirers, slim ladies tends to wannabes, trying to conform to the social standard. This set of slim ladies sometimes goes beyond the radar looking for that thick body physique, consuming all sorts in the name of 'supplements' and drinking only-God-knows various kinds of grassy concoction.

In a world where celebrities edit and photoshop their pictures to achieve that thick body physique, the Hustle to achieve this body type is surreal, people undergo all sorts of diet programs, even their body system becomes confused over the years; to achieve that spec you long wish for, respecting your genes and bodily reactions to the food, stress and 'enjoyment' is one big step in understanding what intuitive eating really means. Despite the fact that intuitive eating is not a dieting plan nor a weight loss program, interestingly, some people have recorded significant loss in weight on commencement of intuitive eating. In respecting your body, sometimes what is good for the goose is not at all times good for the gander. It's okay to have body goals, but don't set unrealistic goals that are not fine-tuned to your body makeup. The essence of intuitive eating is to enable you to achieve that 'bodily homeostasis.' Your hormones know when you crave ice cream and when you crave lemonade, without looking at a Food calendar or timetable.

In some cases, an individual may add weight, and later on, lose weight; this phenomenon is common amongst people whose parents are a mixture of body times and whose 'ancestral body blueprint' is one better described as the best of the two universes. These set of individuals can achieve body goals without necessarily dieting but understanding what redisposes them to weight loss or weight gain. I have heard some people say they lose weight after being exposed to much stress, and shockingly, another group says they add weight when they are stressed. There's no general rule to body reaction to external stimuli. It is not out of place to say one's Man's positive catalyst is another man's negative catalyst. Interestingly some folks say they add weight after days of long hours of sleep; this, however, is not the case with everybody.

Knowing your body and respecting your body, makes you enjoy your intuitive eating journey as you are almost not body about eating your favorite dish every day, even if it is one high in calorie. Intuitive eating boosts self-estimate and improves overall psychological well-being as there is no guilt after taking a bowl of ice cream after having some fries. Just because everyone says, high-calorie foods make one add weight does not mean you will spontaneously add weight after consuming some fried chicken wings.

For example if you suddenly added a few pounds of weight maybe after a vacation somewhere nice, for a body type that is not naturally the chubby type, a few exercises may be actually brought back that body without necessarily changing your diet or creating a few diets, this is more like giving yourself a realistic goal because you comprehend your body type and you respect your body. However, for a person who has born chubby into a chubby family and probably has chubby relatives, trying to hit the gym to achieve a slim physique but sounds like mission impossible, even if it becomes mission - accomplished, it surely cannot be maintained because you have not respected your body, you have just tried to squeeze a football into your trouser pocket - this is how illogical some of the body goals look and sound like without proper understanding of your genetic history and make up the extent that your body is concerned. Many times, I have met men in the gym who are ardent gym-goers who don't go bigger than they have been for months even after religiously hitting the gym, while there are some that within months are growing 'out of proportion' without using steroids.

This further proves that your genetic makeup is important when postulating body goals, and eventually, it boils down to accepting who you are and respecting your body. The idea of Intuitive eating and by extension the philosophy as a whole cannot be valid without obeying or following this eighth principle, because if this principle is not understood and followed, there is a high probability to revert back to dieting because of societal standards, cultural norms and beliefs, and other anti-intuitive eating factors.

This idea of intuitive eating can be likened to a factory reset mode, whereby your mind, thoughts, and standards as far as eating is concerned is a "tabula Raza", that is, a clean slate, here you pick what you want to be written on it, you eat like a kid but not necessarily like a kid, you go for what you want (sometimes even if what you crave is 'junk food', it is all part of the intuitive eating), eat without guilt like a teenager taking chocolate bars. Just like a mobile phone that has been of use for months or years, it definitely has a pattern or memory, starting afresh after a factory reset will definitely not be a smooth ride and nor is the first period after the starting of intuitive eating, the guilts and caution will creep in involuntary, but with time your body and minds get accustomed to the philosophy and not the diet because intuitive eating ib not a dieting type or plan but a philosophy that promotes natural craving and hunger-induced selection of food based on history and personal awareness.

Respecting your body does not just allow intuitive eating to go smooth but the concomitantly improves self-esteem, self-love and in turn create a chain reaction that is capable of breaking societal expectations and standards of body shape, type, and physique that pushes some group off the edge, promotes depression and creating man-made, society-made anti-social individuals. A good way of starting the fruitful journey of respecting your body is;

- Stop comparing yourself with anyone not even celebrities
- Stop typing to be who you see on social media

A good number is a product of Dr 90210 and a professional photoshop work, and for the ones that do not just smile back and be your own crush for starters because if you don't respect your body first, who will? Also remember the reward is not to achieve weight loss but the utmost of all, Love, can we truly love without respect?. How best can we respect if not by first understanding, understand your body, understand that just because you and your roommate eat the same food doesn't mean you two will react accordingly or maintain the same physique. To really enjoy and practice intuitive eating, respecting your body cannot be overstressed. Next time you see a body type you appreciate, if it is one achievable good, and if not, just respect your body and enjoy who you are, remember there was no standard, the standards were made by people like you, be your own standard while striving to be a better you without losing yourself in the process, remember if there is no respect it is not healthy enough and cannot be sustained.

Chapter 14: The Ninth Principle: Exercise- Feel the Difference

The era of militant exercise should be kept aside. Just get active and feel the difference. But, exercise is a unique little something many individuals have various sentiments about. A few people loathe it; a few people endure it; a few people love it. Also, it appears to be distinct for everyone. Notwithstanding, you can Shift your focus to how it feels to move your body, rather than the calorie-burning effect of exercise. If you center around how you feel from working out, such as energized, it can have the effect between turning up for an energetic morning walk or hitting the rest caution. On the off chance that when you wake up, your lone objective is to get in shape, it's typically not a persuading factor at that occasion.

You reclaim satisfaction in eating with the help of intuitive eating syndrome, so it also helps you reclaim satisfaction in movement the way you exercise. At the point when you move in a manner that brings happiness or aliveness, you are genuinely supporting the body, brain, and soul. All bodies are distinct, and everybody appreciates various exercises. Try not to contrast yourself as well as other people; find what works best for you and your extraordinary, valuable body!

Moving ahead, to put this principle into action, I employ you to pen the activities that you enjoy or that you would like to try. Do you feel burly and engaged after a yoga class, a climb in the forested areas, a walk around the recreation center, or riding your bicycle? Don't hesitate to get imaginative here! Shouldn't something be said about ping-pong, volleyball?

Unfortunately to some people, they mistrusted what they felt from exercising with diet culture. If you have to net in shape, it's often advised to go on a diet and start exercising- usually intensely. Entire schedule and advertising efforts in the health business are worked around what number of calories you can consume in a specific exercise or what number of pounds you'll lose if you do this multi-day "fat-consuming" program, for instance. What's more, much the same as slimming down, practicing seriously for a while may award you some weight-loss results; however, it will be short-lived and most likely impossible to sustain in the long-haul.

Weight loss cannot be guaranteed through exercising if that's your sole aim, eventually you are sorely disappointed, and in the end, you will give up prematurely and also miss out on all the great interior and exterior medical benefits of physical activity.

Just like Larry Pupe, who had four different group exercise certifications, and also became a group fitness instructor at the age of 19 years old. One could imagine and asked, how did he attain all this worthiness? Simple, just his passion for exercise cycling in particular. Hey! Did I miss something or omitted it? Here's the thing, if you head straight to the gym because you feel like you 'HAVE TO' rather than because you 'WANT TO', then you're not going to benefit mentally or physically your body will tell you when it needs to work out, and it will give you the desire to do so, but if you would prefer not to, DONT start eating intuitively, bag some days off of the gym if you don't want to go, and as soon as you 'ACTUALLY WANT TO', go to the gym, and see how it feels you will feel a difference, you will should have the option to affix with your body, and truly experience that mind-body connection, rather than going through the motions so are you ready to actually feel good working out? Don't make a schedule. For Larry, all he does at the gym was to tread me with utmost good faith or let say a partial substitute for cycling. Proceeding to the next phase of how to put this principle into play is How might the quest for these exercises sway your life? It may challenge to few who embark on the journey of excitement but the, in the long run, having a negative association with the exercise, this could arise as a result of the reasons to mention a few:

- **Exercise Program with Less Body Fuel:**

The actually happen if you are dieting, and therefore abstaining yourself calories or carbohydrates, it's apparent you may not feel enough drive in your body when exercising, and therefore, it seems to feel like you are pushing yourself to complete the activity. This is not sound nor delightful ways to complete your exercise. Surprisingly, I walk down to a nearby mall after my evening class to get a nice outfit for my gala night, a guy opposite hanger for perfume, and the like was bitterly brunchy on his performance at the gym that it was a total waste of time. Did I think to myself, why the complaint? What could be the course? Suddenly, he saves me the stress; he said, well, actually, I am on diet therapy. Then I concluded within a microsecond that guy suffers from less energy.

Keep in mind, consolidating satisfactory rest is similarly as significant with regards to supportable and feeding self-care! For certain people, the huge practice will take a vacation day from moving your body, when you are feeling worn out, wiped out, or sore. Finally, you might notice some times when your body doesn't feel like moving — and that's okay too. You don't need to acquire rest! Exercise isn't a commitment, and once in a while, the best thing you can accomplish for your wellbeing is to sleep. Be free; your body comprehends what it needs!

Chapter 15: The Tenth Principle: Honor Your Health with Gentle Nutrition

For everything that has a beginning must surely have an end part. But there is nothing like a Happy ending. It's simply in the wake of going on the adventure through the initial nine principles, which assist us with working through unfortunate considerations towards nourishment and ourselves, that we land here — the last principle standing However, I have come to understand that if don't have a solid association with nourishment, eating invigoratingly will be troublesome and may really accomplish more damage than anything else, at last, no stable wellbeing. So, it's crucial you solve the relationship with your food, mind, and body first. You were surprised I made mention of food. Why? A hungry stomach is an angry fellow. Now you can picture why food came out top at the billboard.

Settle on nourishment decisions that respect your wellbeing and taste buds while making you feel well. Remember that you don't have to eat an ideal eating regimen to be sound. You won't all of a sudden get a supplement lack dependent on one tidbit, one dinner, or one day. It's what you eat reliably after some time that counts – progress; not flawlessness is what matters. However, nutrition is important to consider when choosing food. A banana has an unexpected dietary benefit in comparison to a Snickers bar — I could never deny that. However, unbending, high contrast thinking can harm our emotional wellness and association with our bodies… and that is the reason it's about delicate nourishment.

Think about this mantra:

"In issues of taste, think about nourishment; in issues of sustenance, think about taste."

We don't need to bargain for one to have the other. And we can swing excessively far one way — picking things just dependent on taste, and picking things just dependent on nourishment. There is plenty of nourishment info out there, yet this is an incredible spot to begin. The adventure to finding which nourishments respect your wellbeing is continuous, as you tune in lecture while in the classroom, this yet in addition tune in to the messages your body sends you as you have encounters eating various nourishments and noticing how they make you feel.

Gentle sustenance will enable you to seek after wellbeing without feeling like your incentive as an individual relies upon it, and without making you feel denied, on the grounds that all nourishments still fit! In case you have experienced this voyage, you presently get the opportunity to begin filling your body in a manner that really delivers essentialness and life as a top priority, body, and soul. What's more, that is the thing that natural eating is about.

These are general recommendations from dietitians. Everyone needs to feel great, right? To have vitality, no a throbbing painfulness, to deal with yourself. That is so crucial! Along these lines, here are little commonsense ways that you can. Once more, this is a free guideline. Don't follow it exactly, take out any steps that don't jive with you and add in something that does. Start with 1 or 2 of them or better still, Start with all. Do what works best for you, because, at the end of the day, no one knows your body as you do!

Once more, you don't need to turn these suggestions into strict rules. Maybe the cream vanilla harms your stomach; at that point, don't eat it. You can pick the ones that vibe directly for you and even include your own. I will also add briefly, "Honor Your Health" also means that if you have a medical condition or allergy that restricts certain foods, you respect those needs, of course. For example, if you have Celiac, you will probably feel awful if you eat gluten. So, part of honoring your health would be to eat gluten-free foods. But if that is the case, for example, you can still try to choose gluten-free foods that you enjoy and will satisfy you as well.

I think Tribole and Resch (2012) sum-up this last principle nicely when they say: *"Settle on nourishment decisions that respect your wellbeing and taste buds while making you feel well. Remember that you don't have to eat perfectly to be healthy. You won't abruptly get a supplement lack or put on weight from one tidbit, one supper, or one day of eating. It's what you eat reliably after some time that matters progress; not flawlessness is the thing that matters."*

Chapter 16: Confusion About Nutrition

It's not simply you. Diet science on rudiments like fat, sugar, and salt is confounding by structure. Nutritionists state they can barely go out without somebody asking them for what reason dietary exhortation is so confounding. How could it be that researchers (scientists) can alter human DNA; however, can't state for certain whether fundamental nourishments like nuts and eggs are beneficial for us? Nuts, when thought about too greasy to even think about justifying eating in any noteworthy sum, were restored by discoveries from a huge, long term study that discovered individuals who ate nuts lived longer and were no fatter than the individuals who didn't.

What's more, eggs, when despised for containing an excessive amount of cholesterol, are back on the approval list in the proposed 2015 U.S. dietary recommendations presented in January. The open remark time frame on the recommendations closes one week from now. These aren't the main nourishments whose wellbeing worth is being reevaluated in the new recommendations.

The new proposals invert past perspectives about fat by focusing exactly on soaked fats. They likewise set espresso back on the menu for the wellbeing cognizant set. Better hold the sugar, however. Sustenance science has been portraying a dimmer view of including sugars. The 2015 recommendations present, just because, a top on the amount of our complete caloric admission we can securely get from including sugar. They put that number at about ten percent, which is still twofold what the American Heart Association proposes. "Everyone has a conclusion on sustenance," said Sylvia Rowe, an aide educator and the previous leader of the International Food Information Council. "We all eat. We as a whole have a comprehension of it, however by and large we have values."

There are a few things that make sustenance an intense nut to pop open, logically. For instance, since we all consume an assortment of nourishments, it's difficult for specialists to parse the body's reaction to one explicit nourishment the manner in which they could with a medicine. Furthermore, a specialist can just occasionally legitimize acquiring individuals into a patient setting to control everything else they eat. In most cases, they depend on asking individuals what they ate the day preceding — and individuals frequently don't recollect. Shouldn't something be mentioned about creature studies?

"Creatures are not smaller than normal individuals, they have various ways of life and dietary propensities," said an author of food Politics and professor of nutrition and sociology at New York University. "Coprophagia (a few creatures' propensities for eating each other's crap), for instance, is profoundly frustrating."

How Industry Influences Nutrition Studies

The fundamental issue with nourishment science is by all accounts that nourishment is enormous business, and nourishment combinations impact the inquiries that are posed and the appropriate responses that are given or not. The nourishment business leaves its fingerprints on look into, pundits state, beginning with the way inquire about plans are set, through financing considers prone to swing their direction and jabbing gaps in the examination behind negative discoveries. The business additionally drives the government to rejigger the manner in which it introduces those discoveries as recommendations and overwhelms wellbeing messages with publicizing.

It very well may be difficult to bind precisely what impact the industry has on the state of scientific accord with regards to intriguing issues like sugar and meat. In any case, Kimber Stanhope, Ph.D., a nutritional biologist at the University of California, Davis, has a good vantage point. Stanhope, a sugar experimenter, broadcast an investigation a week ago in the American

Journal of Clinical Nutrition with sensational, and conceivably dubious, discoveries.

The investigation indicated that devouring even a large portion of a soft drink of high-fructose corn syrup (HFCS) with every feast was sufficient to generously build cardiovascular hazard factors in youthful grown-ups. Stanhope uncovered a couple of late investigations that discovered the exact inverse of hers.

In those investigations, even a higher everyday portion of HFCS demonstrated no noteworthy impacts. These investigations were supported with an unhindered award from the Corn Refiners Association, the industry bunch that makes high-fructose corn syrup. The significant author on both of those examinations was Dr. James Rippe, whose work has likewise been supported by ConAgra Foods, PepsiCo International, and Kraft. Stanhope's investigation was financed by the National Institutes of Health (NIH).

The two examinations gave members three sweet refreshments daily, yet were, other than that, very unique. Stanhope and her associates gave sweet Kool-Aid drinks that contained a biomarker that enabled them to confirm that the members were normally drinking the sweet beverages by testing their pee. The control gathering got beverages improved with aspartame. Members in the business supported investigation got their HFCS in low-fat milk. Stanhope said it was an odd decision given that as much as 66% of the populace can't endure lactose. The investigation didn't confirm that members who said they were drinking the milk truly were.

Low-fat milk has also been depicted to improve the very same cardiovascular markers the study was testing. And there was no control group to weed out those effects. In addition, while separating results for men and women is a baseline requirement for most medical journals, Rippe's study didn't sort them out. Also, Stanhope indicated one lot of line diagrams that were made to appear to be identical — demonstrating no impact of HFCS — by utilizing an alternate size of qualities. Rippe didn't react to a solicitation for input. "if you hear the disappointment in my voice, it's because of considering what I could have finished with that cash, the general wellbeing addresses I could help answer," Stanhope said, "Why are we arguing about such basic things?" These dueling studies illustrate a larger problem.

A 2013 examination broadcasted in the journal PLOS Medicine indicated that reviews financed by industry were multiple times as prone to find that there wasn't sufficient proof to close sugar-improved beverages like soda are linked to weight addiction and obesity. Stanhope worries things may get worse rather than better. She thinks about whether she'll ever get the opportunity to bring patients into an emergency clinic setting, as she did toward the start and end of the HFCS study. The NIH has quit taking care of the additional expenses of in-quiet examinations as an approach to cut costs. It trusts industry will take care of everything, which may bode well for pharmaceutical research where the business sells potential fixes, yet not for the nourishment business, where the item is frequently the issue Nutritionists state the absence of government financing for their domain is nearly as large an issue as the nearness of industry investigation. By the method of appraisal, the 2014 innovative work spending plan for a solitary organization, PepsiCo, was half as large as the NIH's whole sustenance spending plan for that year.

Where's the Beef?

Mary Story, Ph.D., RD, the program executive for Healthy Eating Research, was a member of the 2015 dietary recommendation board of trustees. She says there was definitely no industry impact on their recommendations, an assertion Schmidt thinks is likely true.

In any case, a part of the manners in which government proposals take into account industry and at last make disarray might be profoundly installed all the while. "The government has an 'eat increasingly' predisposition," said Katie Ferraro, MPH, RD, a nutritionist at UCSF. The government, and particularly the USDA, whose objective is to help horticulture, is placed in an awkward position if it advises purchasers to eat less of some random item, on the grounds that doing so will hurt the ranchers and agribusinesses that produce the item.

You can see this in prior guidance to pick "lean meats" (with no particular reference to what those might be) or to "limit" as opposed to staying away from sugar. In the 2015 recommendations, for example, there's a push to eat more "plant-based nourishments." "They won't come right out and state, 'Eat fewer dairy animals,'" Ferraro said.

In any case, pushing for plant nourishments is nearer to calling for "fewer dairy animals" than past rules, which upheld for "lean meats." The meat entryway has targeted the more up to date language. Ferraro says she sees the administration moving to more brilliant counsel on fats in the new recommendation. "What they're not saying this time is, 'Pursue a low-fat eating regimen.' What that is basically saying is, 'We were thoroughly off-base.'

What occurred with a low-fat eating routine was everybody put on a lot of weight," she said. The more recent language likewise loses a part of the layers of confusion that accompany discussing supplements like soaked fats as opposed to naming the nourishments — like meat, entire milk, and spread — that we should mostly avoid. "It's professional stability for dieticians," Ferraro gag.

"There is a requirement for a believable expert in translating government doublespeak." But much more clear language would accomplish more to assist Americans with choosing more advantageous nourishments. Some keep on legitimizing potato chips as "plant-based nourishments," for instance. "Individuals don't go to the store to purchase fiber, salt, and potassium. They go to the store to purchase food," Ferraro said. "I'm happy to see (the government) making more nourishment-based suggestions. That's helpful." So what foods should you eat? Every nutritionist Health line addressed said that the Mediterranean eating routine had been known to be best for in any event ten years. The eating regimen incorporates vegetables and common products, vegetables and whole grains, a few nuts and low-fat dairy, some fish and chicken, with little included sugar or red meat, "lean" or something else. Including or subtracting an egg scarcely matters. Espresso or no espresso matters even less.

"Essential dietary counsel continues as before — steady, however dull," Nestle wrote in 2002. Here's another entire confusion about nutrition, which is a myth, Diet Myth. Myth can simply be defined as a thought or story that was advised in an antiquated culture to clarify a practice, belief, or natural occurrence that isn't valid.

Since we know the actual meaning now, we shouldn't give in to the abstracts that seem as facts it brings forth. Almost consistently, another scientific investigation about diet and wellbeing scare head. Staying aware of the most recent nourishment examine - also the recess jabber - can be overwhelming. You might be enticed to surrender in dissatisfaction and return to your old dietary patterns. In any case, don't give nourishment perplexity a chance to keep you from your objectives. Below are some misconceptions about diet and sustenance and the certainties behind them.

Diet Myth No. 1: Carbohydrates make you fat.

Certainty: Carbs have gotten terrible notoriety as far back as Dr. Atkins advised his devotees to maintain a strategic distance from them, thinking back to the '70s. The truth of the matter is that starches don't cause weight increase anything else than proteins or fats do. If you eat a large number of calories - which can just originate from carbs, protein, fat, or liquor - you put on weight. The facts confirm that refined carbs (like sugar and white flour) will, in general, be immediately processed, leaving you hungry again not long after you eat them. Yet, rather than staying away from all carbs, pick brilliant carbs, for example, entire grains, natural products, and vegetables.

Diet Myth No. 2: Dairy nourishments have such a large quantity of calories, and once you have quit developing, who needs dairy items at any rate?

Certainty: You do require increasingly bone-building calcium during dynamic development.

In any case, grown-ups keep on requiring calcium, alongside Vitamin D, for the lifespan of their lives, to keep up the bone structure and to counteract infections, for example, osteoporosis. Furthermore, dairy items are commonly the best root of calcium in the eating routine. It's ideal to pick without fat and low-fat dairy items, for controlling calories, cholesterol, and soaked fat — the U.S.

Department of Agriculture's 2005 Dietary Guidelines prescribes three servings of low-fat or sans fat dairy every day for grown-ups.

Diet Myth No. 3: Eating eggs all the time prompts elevated cholesterol levels.

Certainty: The egg has been recovered. The American Heart Association's dietary recommendation never again make any proposal about what number of egg yolks you ought to eat in seven days. Eggs are an implausible root of protein, B nutrients, iron, and different minerals - all fundamental to wellbeing. One huge egg has just 80 calories and 5 grams, yet is filling enough to keep you fulfilled for a future time. Eggs are flexible, modest, and can be eaten for any dinner of the day. In case you're a solid grown-up, you can appreciate an egg a day without concern.

Diet Myth No. 4: Artificial sugars check your sweet tooth.

Certainty: The advantage of utilizing fake sugars is that you get the sweet taste with no additional calories. Unfortunately, eating and drinking misleadingly improved nourishments just propagates our inborn want for sweetness. Take a stab at fulfilling your sweet tooth with the common sweetness of organic product (solidified natural product, similar to grapes, is particularly fulfilling). Or then again, sprinkle cinnamon or another delightful zest on yogurt for a turn on sweetness. The objective is to gradually lessen your longing for sweet nourishments and beverages rather than essentially substituting those made with fake sugars. If you do appreciate nourishments and refreshments improved with counterfeit sugars, do as such with some restraint.

Diet Myth No. 5: If you eat the greater part of your calories late around evening time, you'll put on weight.

Certainty: The well-known adage, 'Have to breakfast like a lord, lunch like a sovereign, and supper like a poor person" depended on the possibility that since you're increasingly dynamic for the lengthy duration of the day, you ought to eat more when you're destined to consume it off.

In any case, the primary concern for overseeing weight is the hard and fast number of calories you consume during the day. Despite when you eat them, in the event that you take in more than you consume, you will put on weight, and if you take in less, you'll lose. All things considered, remember that evening time eating tends to be fixated on inactive exercises, frequently appearing as thoughtless chomping before the TV. And calories consumed during the night will, in general, be "extra" calories, as opposed to required ones. That is the reason many eating routine specialists suggest closing down the kitchen after supper.

Diet Myth No. 6: You can eat all the sans fat nourishments you like without putting on weight.

Certainty: sans fat nourishments are not sans calorie food sources, and they consider some portion of your day's calorie assignment. At the point when without fat nourishments were presented, numerous individuals disregarded controlling bit size and ate as quite a bit of these nourishments as they needed - at that point, asked why they weren't getting more fit! Peruse the names and check the recorded bit size to decide how without fat nourishments can fit into your eating plan. Moreover, nourishments that are tagged as being "trans fats free" are not free of calories. They may even contain some trans fats; makers are permitted to mark a nourishment "trans-fat-free" when it has up to 0.5 grams of trans fats per serving. Your most logical option is to check the rundown of fixings to check whether there are any in part hydrogenated fats in the nourishment. Sometimes, producers have supplanted trans fats with soaked fats or different, not exactly solid fixings.

Diet Myth No. 7: It's an impractical notion to nibble between suppers.

Certainty: Snacks can be a piece of any sound eating routine, as long as you pick them shrewdly. A considerable number of don't have such numerous optional calories to save in their weight control plans, so go for tidbits that give some solid supplements, similar to natural products, vegetables, low-fat dairy items, and low-fat popcorn. What's more, watch part measures - a sensible tidbit is one that is under 200 calories.

Diet Myth No. 8: Peanut spread is definitely not sturdy nourishment.

Certainty: Peanut margarine is high in fat and frequently high in sodium; however, it additionally contains much more sound unsaturated fats than immersed fats. At the point when you eat soaked fats with some restraint, and generally pick unsaturated fats, you can help lower LDL "awful" cholesterol and diminish your danger of coronary illness. Peanut butter is additionally great root of fiber (particularly stout nutty spread), and potassium, which is deficient in numerous American weight control plans It even has a spot in weight reduction diets; thinks about have indicated that a little part can keep you feeling filled for a considerable length of time.

How to Handle Ever-Changing or Misguided Information About Nutrition?

It appears as if nourishment news is consistently evolving Official recommendations say one thing regarding what to eat, however, diet books and bloggers may offer diverse counsel frequently to expel sound nourishments from your eating routine for no tenable explanation. In case you are confounded about the right sustenance information to pursue, you're not alone. It can make you wonder, is nutrition science worth listening to at all? Never mind, misguided information about nutrition could simply be handled by the following ways:

What to Study

Foods contain zillions of mixes. At the point when sustenance scientists endeavor to associate nourishment to sickness, they frequently don't know which segment of the nourishment to think about. For instance, we realize that eating developed starting from the earliest decrease's malignant growth. However, what parts are malignancy defensive?

Food Affects Our Health in various Ways and Diverse Ages

For instance, if pregnant (or thinking of), you may be afraid to eat fish in fear the mercury in fish will damage your baby. Yet, fish contains the prime root of the omega-3 fats that are essential for optimal brain development in the fetus. Absorbing too little DHA (of a kind of omega-3 fat) can add to irreversible mental health issues. With the creature considers, a low admission of DHA results in more slow mind development, consideration issues, impulsivity, and critical thinking aptitudes. With human investigations that supplement the maternal eating regimen with DHA, the infants adapt quicker and recollect information better.

When the children have arrived at age four, these advantages convert into higher IQs. What's more, by age five, longer supported consideration. In case you have been frightened off from eating fish as a result of dread of mercury harming, you ought to make certain to take a gander at the entire picture, regardless of whether you are a lady examining pregnancy or a maturing competitor needing to lessen the danger of coronary illness (fish eaters have less heart disease.)

The prescribed absorption is to adore DHA-rich fish, for example, pink salmon once every week- - in spite of conceivable mercury content- - and another 6 oz. every seven day stretch of low-mercury fish and shellfish (shrimp, crab, scallops, light fish, pollock).

A Poor Diet Takes Years to Unfold

As a youthful competitor in your 20s and 30s, you may think you are impenetrable and insusceptible from coronary illness. Maybe you eat anything you desire, regardless of whether it's omelets or pepperoni pizza. And you likely feel fine (today). In any case, if your "see nourishment" diet (you eat what you see) prompts elevated cholesterol in your mid-age, you will have a greater danger of declining mental status as you age.

Arteries obstructed with cholesterol and immersed fat lead to cardiovascular malady, yet in addition to dementia and Alzheimer's.

The more you live, the higher your danger of dementia. While just a single percent of 60-year-olds have dementia, 40 percent of 90-year-olds do. gosh! What would you be able to do to anticipate dementia? Appreciate more products of the vegetable and fish (two times every week). What is useful for your heart is also useful for your brain!

Don't crash-diet to shed fat quickly! You'll lose a lot of muscle. These outcomes in a less-sound body in light of the fact that your wellbeing relies upon your strength load. For ideal wellbeing and weight, do quality training programs to assemble muscle and eat just a little less around evening time to lose fat.

Notices

Ads for nutrient enhancements and medications make light of the significance of diet and exercise. Consequently, pills and powerful meds appear to be more compelling than eating well and exercising regularly.

Too hardly any individuals understand that activity is the best way to deal with to improve by and large wellbeing and insusceptible reaction, especially as we age. No disarray about this: If your folks, as well as grandparents, carry on with an inactive way of life, let them realize they should go for an everyday stroll (ideally to the exercise center). Research demonstrates mice who practiced normally had quicker injury mending, better endurance of influenza and infections, and less aggravation. Fit older individuals experience comparable advantages. For kids and grown-ups the same, eating great to fuel a functioning way of life is without question a significant key to deep-rooted wellbeing and life span!

Chapter 17: Scientists Thoughts on Intuitive Eating

In this chapter, there are many scientific research and thoughts towards intuitive eating in various ways. A few of the thought is discussed here on balancing nutrition with intuitive eating, the study of the eating regimen on which food is off-limits, and science behind careful eating.

Balancing Nutrition with Intuitive Eating

There has been somewhat of a dialog of late that supporting natural eating and wellbeing at each size is proportionate to giving the center finger to great nourishment. I'm here to guarantee you that couldn't in any way be off-base. Kicking diets to the control, finishing limitation, and grasping genuine nourishment opportunity enables you to improve your sustenance without all the blame and insane principles consuming fewer calories makes. You likewise get the chance to grasp sustenance from the point of view of mending your association with nourishment.

key Nutrition Is Balance Over Time

First, key nourishment is an exercise in careful control. It isn't highly contrasting. Our needs vary contingent upon our activity levels, hereditary qualities, age, sexual orientation, feelings of anxiety, and a large number of other wellbeing conditions that change our requirements for fundamental nourishment. This change is typical, and a completely scripted feast plan will never represent these varieties. Natural eating does. When you figure out how to tune in to your body signals, you figure out how to differ your nourishment absorption dependent on your individual needs. Have you at any point had a hankering for more protein, or perhaps a major bowl of pasta? That is your body's method for saying, "Hello, young lady; I need somewhat more of… ".

Indeed even the most experienced professionals realize we generally need to burrow somewhat more profound. Lab work enables us to do only that. Estimating your cholesterol, triglycerides, blood glucose, irritation markers, supplement status, and hormone levels gives a much more clear picture of how your body is functioning than weight alone. The great news is taking lab estimations enables you to utilize nourishment science as an apparatus to help your body rather than a weapon utilized against it. Labs can work connected at the hip with a natural eating practice. Envision this, you have your labs drawn, and we discover your cholesterol is high, and your blood glucose is raised into pre-diabetic reaches. Utilizing natural eating, we would discover nourishments you really like and anticipate eating while simultaneously improving your blood markers. You figure out how to turn out to be more on top of your body signals. This empowers you to gorge less on nourishments you recently dreaded and kept beyond reach until you couldn't bear it anymore. You end the cycle of yo-yo eating fewer carbs that exacerbates your blood markers each time you lose and put on weight. You discover balance in eating once more. **Food Can Remove the Stress of satisfying Nutrient Needs.**

Utilizing supplements in a decent and supplement thick diet isn't something I avoid. While I generally need you to expand your nourishment through the food sources you eat, I additionally comprehend that enhancements can assume a key job in natural eating. When you're figuring out how to tune in to your body again, they assist you with meeting your nutrient and mineral needs, enabling you to drop the pressure of hitting macros and macros when picking nourishments. When picking supplements, an individualized methodology is in every case best. There's an examination (truly cool research as I would see it) that shows supplementation can help with interminable conditions like diabetes, weakness, sorrow, coronary illness, joint pain, and a scope of different conditions.

Diets for weight reduction ordinarily include confinement. The 5:2 eating regimen depends on confining calories, and the ketogenic diet depends on limiting specific sorts of nourishment.

However, explore recommends that prohibitive abstaining from excessive food intake can prompt a higher weight file (BMI) after some time and a more prominent future probability of being overweight. There is likewise proof recommending that nourishment confinement can prompt a distraction with nourishment, coerce about eating, and more significant levels of wretchedness, uneasiness, and stress. So, if diets don't generally assist you with shedding pounds and could add to mental issues, what different arrangements are there? As of late, there has been an expanded spotlight on the idea of "intuitive eating."

Intuitive eating was made known by two dietitians, Evelyn Tribole and Elyse Resch, who authored a book regarding the matter and built up a site devoted to the subject. The objective of eating naturally is to tune in to your body and enable it to direct you on when and the amount to eat, as opposed to being impacted by your condition, feelings, or the principles endorsed by eats fewer carbs. The idea is like careful eating, and the terms are frequently utilized reciprocally. Mindful eating includes building up the consciousness of inward craving and satiety cues and settling on cognizant nourishment decisions.

It underlines the significance of focusing on the enthusiastic and physical sensations experienced while eating. In contrast to numerous different weight control plans, instinctive eating urges you to eat what you want; no food is off-limits. While some may anticipate that this should prompt eating all the more high-fat or high-sugar nourishments, investigation recommends this isn't the situation. Upholder of natural eating proposes that the more you confine yourself, the almost certain you are to gorge later. The idea of natural eating is straightforward and doesn't include confounded dietary standards. But what does the proof recommend?

Beneficial outcome on Mental Health

As far as weight reduction, it isn't yet evident that natural eating is more compelling than calorie confinement. Results from observational examinations found that individuals who ate naturally had a lower BMI than the individuals who didn't. Be that as it may, since individuals who confine may do so in light of the fact that they as of now have a high BMI, it is hard to decide the genuine impact natural eating had. Also, results from intercession contemplate with overweight or corpulent individuals are not as clear. For example, one instance found that of the eight investigations assessed, only two noted a reduction in weight from intuitive eating.

In a later survey, weight reduction was seen in just eight out of 16 investigations. Also, out of the eight, weight reduction was measurably critical in just three. Unlike different eating regimens, the central point of natural eating isn't on weight reduction yet rather on tending to the reasons why individuals eat. In this way, regardless of whether its viability as a weight reduction strategy is dubious, it could at present give benefits by advancing smart dieting conduct.

This plausibility has been upheld by research recommending natural eating may prompt a decrease in voraciously consuming food indications and eating for outer and passionate reasons. Natural eating is additionally connected with more direct positive self-perception, body fulfillment, positive, enthusiastic working, and higher self-esteem.

Finally, an ongoing report found that more significant levels of natural eating anticipated lower dietary problem manifestations, contrasted and calorie-checking, and visit self-gauging. This is a difference to normal prohibitive eating less junk food, which has been related to an expanded danger of scattered eating, one that might be more prominent for the people who additionally experience manifestations of despondency and low confidence. While more research should be led to build up if natural eating can prompt weight reduction, the beneficial outcomes on emotional wellness and smart dieting conduct are promising. One issue with natural eating is that it expects we can precisely tell how ravenous or full we are. Research recommends that individuals who are better at seeing inner sensations may likewise eat all the more naturally.

However, since there is proof that individuals with dietary issues experience issues perceiving signals from inside their body, it appears to be conceivable that a few people may battle to react to the natural eating approach basically in light of the fact that they battle to tune in to their very own bodies. Likewise, while it appears to be consistent just to eat dependent on inward sensations as opposed to natural prompts, for some individuals, this is certainly not a viable remedy.

The time at which we eat, for example, adhering to explicit family tea-time, or assigned occasions during work to have a mid-day break is often out of our control. While on a fundamental level, eating when you are eager appears to be perfect, by and by, it isn't constantly conceivable. Natural eating might be a compelling method to get in shape, however so far there isn't sufficient proof to propose that it works superior to customary, calorie-prohibitive weight control plans. However, the advantages to mental wellbeing that eating naturally gives propose it is a considerably more solid approach to plan with how we eat. It may not work for everybody, especially the individuals who battle to feel sensations in their own bodies. Be that as it may, when it appears that everything in our condition is revealing to us what to eat and the amount to eat, it might merit setting aside some effort to tune in to your body to discover what you need.

How Do Mindfulness-Based Interventions Relate to Mindful Eating?

Research studies utilizing MBIs to prepare a person to take care of their eating practices without judgment have varied from concentrate to consider. Instances of these intercessions incorporate utilizing an answer scale from "never/once in a while" to "ordinarily/consistently" to pass on prompts, for example, "When a café segment is excessively huge, I quit eating when I'm full" or "I nibble without seeing I am eating."

In spite of the slight contrasts in mediations, the objectives of these investigations stay reliable: to distinguish whether care and additionally careful eating aptitudes may improve unfortunate eating practices. While there is no single e

03ndless supply of careful eating, the writer recommends that it by and largely utilizes at least one of the accompanying:

- Mindfully taking care of the eating background by seeing the smell, surface, and taste of the nourishment

- Reducing the speed of eating

- Acknowledging reactions to nourishment (preferences, abhorrence's, or impartial) without judgment

- Becoming mindful of a physical craving and satiety signs to direct your choices to start and finish eating

Research on Mindful Eating and Effects on Eating Behaviors

Though explore the viability of MBIs on eating practices is still generally new, the outcomes have been promising. Several investigations have inspected the impacts of utilizing MBIs on the occurrence of voraciously consuming food, enthusiastic eating, outer eating, and weight put on or weight support.

Binge Eating

Two writing surveys on care-based mediations found that these intercessions diminished the occurrence of pigging out scenes. These outcomes were most grounded when care-based mediations explicitly tended to eat practices and were joined with psychological conduct treatments (which include figuring out how to change unhelpful reasoning examples and additionally practices). It's significant that outcomes didn't improve when the mediation utilized a general care-based pressure decrease (MBSR) program without including substance identified with eating practices.

Passionate Eating

A deliberate survey found that enthusiastic eating improved over most of the concentrates that focused on this eating conduct. Another survey discovered comparative outcomes aside from when they contained members who were not enrolled for enthusiastic eating concerns and additionally detailed low degrees of passionate eating at the pattern. For the most part, the MBIs were best when they included both a careful eating intercession and a subjective social acknowledgment mediation. Those with just the MBSR didn't measurably fundamentally improve passionate eating results.

External Eating

Findings from a writing survey on careful eating, care, and natural eating show that care can help diminish outside eating by lessening the responsiveness of people to outer signals, for example, engaging nourishment bundling or promotions and time of day. This survey likewise recommended that careful eating procedures are best when combined with acknowledgment strategies.

Weight Gain or Weight Maintenance

The accessible proof on care and weight reduction recommend that care preparing alone, without supplemental conduct weight the board methodologies or direction, may not deliver noteworthy or steady weight reduction. Additionally, most investigations have not been surveyed longer than a couple of months, so long term impacts of weight presently can't seem to be considered.

Restrictions, Summary and Future Discussions

The impact of care put together mediations with respect to undesirable eating practices is empowering. Regardless, it's important that there were impediments to these surveys. Huge numbers of the investigations had distinctive objective populaces and utilized various mediations. Additionally, the examination members would, in general, be fundamentally the same as in sexual orientation, ethnicity, and age: most were white, grown-up females. The consequences of these examinations warrant further research and follow-up on the more extended term impacts of MBIs. In spite of these confinements, these discoveries add to the developing proof that care and careful eating can improve undesirable eating practices.

Chapter 18: Putting Intuitive Diet into Practice

Not to be documented under the 'New Year, New You' saying, intuitive eating is utilized to recover a solid association with nourishment that is totally economical – not at all like most diet patterns and health trends. With a plan to make harmony with our nourishment and expel poisonous self-disgracing, this mind-body approach is developing in notoriety and feels exceptionally fundamental in our hyper-associated 'offer and look at' computerized world.

To get why, and how to apply it to your life, we solicited intuitive eating mentor and organizer from Rooted Living, Pandora Paloma, to clarify all. For what reason is intuitive eating so applicable today?

"On the planet, we live in now with #fitspo, superfoods and trend eat less, it's getting increasingly hard to comprehend what genuine wellbeing is. We are moving further and further away from confiding in our very own bodies to give us the sign of when to eat when to back off when to rest. There is a lot of what I call 'clamor' in the health world, yet we shouldn't generally accept the promotion. If diets worked, we wouldn't have 66% of Brits on an eating routine at some random time.

My natural eating and living work consider your enthusiastic express, your association with nourishment, your attitudes, and how your internal pundit is giving orders. It considers your association with yourself and your fulfillment in life outside of nourishment. We're living in a period where we're more associated with others than any time in recent memory, yet I accept we've lost association with ourselves – and our bodies – thus. Genuine wellbeing needs to begin with your life and confiding in your body and mentality. I accept that when you change your life, you change your association with nourishment, your psyche, and your body."

How can it advantage individuals who have issues with nourishment and self-perception? "Regardless of whether you tally calories, have a fixation on being 'sound,' have attempted each diet under the sun or have issues with enthusiastic eating, instinctive eating can assist you with understanding your passionate express, your eating regimen attitudes and how you can fix your association with nourishment. It gives you a rule and backing. You can't simply rip the eating regimen culture mortar off, or you'll be left with an open injury. Rather, by working with the procedure of instinctive eating and living, you can begin stripping back each layer close by building the following, which arrives in a progression of help and proficiency to address whatever side effects or issues you are confronting. I myself have serious issues with nourishment and my body; thus, I realize direct how controlling and overpowering it can feel. You need to open up all that you've been persuaded about nourishment and how your body 'should' look, and re-arrange it with a progressively sympathetic methodology. You also decipher how to manufacture trust in your body. We each realize our bodies superior to any other individual; however, the mind-body association frequently goes somewhat amiss."

What Are Your Top Tips for Rehearsing Natural Eating?

1. **Acknowledge Convenient Solution Prevailing Fashions and Advertising**

"It's enticing to accept that there's a method to get more fit rapidly, effectively and forever by taking extreme measures, taking out whole nutrition types, profoundly cutting calories or going on a low-carb diet. In any case, truly, a great many people can't supersede their body's normal science and longings for expanded timeframes.

Rather than attempting diet after diet just to feel like a disappointment each time you tumble off the wagon, quit eating less junk food altogether. Basic. Surrender the possibility that there are new and better diets prowling around the bend and come back to what has worked for individuals for a considerable length of time: eating genuine nourishments, rehearsing control, and moving your body! Go for a thick supplement diet that supports a sound body, stable personality, and enduring vitality levels, all without attempting to be 'impeccable.'

Settle on nourishment decisions that respect your wellbeing and fulfill your taste buds, while likewise making you feel great from the back to front."

1. **Fuel Yourself with Enough Calories**

when we deny the assemblage of calories, it can make the body store fat so as to endure "The objective of weight reduction shouldn't become the dominant focal point, yet rather be taken care of as a second thought to concentrate on general wellbeing and feeling great in your body.

The inspiration of basically needing to get more fit to look better, particularly for a particular occasion, for example, an occasion or wedding, can be brief and momentary, however significantly more critically, it makes numerous individuals deny themselves of enough calories and rest, which effectively affects the digestion. Perceive that it's imperative to give your body the calories it needs, else you're probably going to manage sentiments of low vitality, hardship, and disdain, or the inclination to gorge or gorge because of natural changes."

1. **Avoid 'Great'/'Awful' Nourishments. Think About A Nourishment You Think About Awful. Why?**

While the facts demonstrate that a few nourishments are more supplement thick than others, vowing to dispose of specific nourishments or nutrition types from your eating regimen perpetually can simply build pressure and sentiments of pre-occupation with those taboo food sources. Natural eating plans to makes harmony with nourishment considers a détente and stops the nourishment battle between your gut and your mind! I frequently find that when you reveal to yourself that you can't or shouldn't have specific nourishment until kingdom come, it can prompt extraordinary sentiments of disgrace alongside wild desires.

This 'win big, or bust' pondering nourishments possibly improves the probability for gorging in light of the fact that when you at last surrender to this taboo nourishment, you are very enticed to eat enormous sums, to feel like it's the last possibility. This normally just expedites further sentiment of blame.

1. **Learn to Eat When You're Eager and Stop When You Are Full**

Become acquainted with what it feels like to be easily full without being excessively stuffed.

In instinctive eating, we utilize a craving scale, which encourages you to distinguish when you are under-or indulging. Make an effort not to get 'hangry' as this effectively lead to indulging before arriving at satiety just as playing destruction with your glucose levels.

1. **Be Cognizant**

Numerous individuals think that its supportive to back off when eating, bite nourishment well, eat undistracted (not working, staring at the TV, driving, and so forth.), and to delay in a dinner or tidbit to take note of how full they feel.

1. **Learn the Distinction Among Fulfillment and Completion**

There is a major distinction in feeling full and feeling fulfilled. Inquire as to whether what you're having is really fulfilling you, or in case you're just eating it since it's there. If you don't cherish it, don't eat it, and if you love it, relish it!

Find ways to tackle pressure.

1. **What Are Your Present Ways of Dealing with Stress or What New Systems Would You Be Able to Utilize?**

I can't reveal to you what number of my customers eat through fatigue! We as a whole vibe intense feelings; disappointment, nervousness, dejection, or weariness; however, understand that nourishment can't really fix any of these emotions or take care of issues throughout your life.

Enthusiastic eating may feel great at the time, yet it quite ends up exacerbating the underlying issue even, on the grounds that then you need to manage sentiments of disgrace or inconvenience, as well. Find different approaches to decrease pressure or fatigue by considering how you feel fulfilled? This is a major piece of my program as nourishment is never more often than not the issue with cluttered eating. I generally look outside of this with customers to perceive how they are staying aware of bliss and fulfillment."

1. **Practice Body Acknowledgment**

At the point when you quit attempting to arrive at the dream body that may never occur, you can begin to dope out how to adore your body as it is presently. Much the same as there is no ideal eating routine, there is no ideal body. At the point when you love your body, you unravel how to support it from within."

There you have it all the different ways to actually get accustomed to the practical aspect of the intuitive diet.

Once again, these guidelines give room for innovation i.e. if you if are aware that something is actually working well for that is out these recommendations, I suggest you keep it up and see you at the next level.

Conclusion

Here's a quick review of Intuitive Eating; Intuitive eating sounds so simple that it's hard to believe it can assist you in maintaining a healthy weight: Eat what you want, however, just when you feel hungry and quit eating when you feel full. Intuitive eating was characterized about 25 years prior by two enlisted dieticians—Evelyn Tribole, MS, RDN, CEDRD-S, and Elyse Resch, MS, RDN, CEDRD-S. They describe intuitive eating less by what it is as by what it isn't. It's anything but an "eat-this-not-that" sort of diet. It isn't even an eating routine, at any rate not in a similar shape as the Grapefruit Diet, the Atkins Diet, the South Beach Diet, or any of those. Actually, it's a greater amount of an enemy of diet. You don't tally calories. You don't wipe out specific nourishment.

You don't pursue any calendar, table, or program as indicated by Tribole and Resch; intuitive eating is a response to "diet culture and weight fixation." "There is genuinely not an isolated long-term study that shows that weight reduction eating fewer carbs is maintainable. Many examinations show that eating less junk food and nourishment limitation with the end goal of weight reduction prompts more weight gain," Tribole documented on their site. "Worse the attention and distraction on weight prompts body disappointment and weight shame, which contrarily impacts wellbeing."

Its originators make it extremely evident that intuitive eating isn't proposed to be a weight reduction strategy. Rather, they depict it as a "weight-impartial model." You may not get in shape; however, natural eating shouldn't make you put on weight, either. Good healthful propensities and a reasonable eating regimen aren't created in one day, nor are they obliterated in one uneven feast. Stimulating eating implies a way of life of settling on decisions and choices, arranging, and realizing how to soothe on speedy and insightful decisions when you haven't arranged. What you find out about eating in these first years all alone will help set up great dietary examples for an incredible remainder. Making the break from home cooking and getting to be liable for picking the nourishments you to eat is a piece of the test of turning into development and an autonomous grown-up.

Ten years back, my cholesterol level at long last hit an edge that my primary care physician could allude me to a pro for help with my eating issues. First stop, a nutritionist. The nutritionist concurs that I need more help than she can offer, so we audit a rundown of centers, advisors, and specialists having some expertise in dietary problems Some of the spots have year-long holding up records. I can't hang tight this long for help. So, I consider a specialist that runs a gathering treatment program in Toronto; we meet and examine my eating history. This was the point at which I originally learned of the intuitive eating development.

After a couple of individual sessions, I joined an open-finished psychotherapy gathering. I prefer not to let it be known; however, I don't recall much about the substance or format of the gathering treatment sessions. I think we commenced every session talking about how our eating went adhering to the intuitive eating rules. Later on, we discussed our feelings, circumstances, nourishment, and eating, endeavoring to stick point the explanations behind our individual issues.

Sometimes we had an action; something to reinforce your mental self-portrait. We shut the session with some kind of feel-great custom.

Thinking back, there were two primary issues with gathering (from my point of view) treatment:

1. Despite being a piece of this gathering for in any event a half year, I didn't totally comprehend the intuitive eating rules, explicitly, eat what your body needs. You would imagine that in the wake of partaking in a gathering for this timeframe, I would realize that your body needs sound nourishments, and it's your mind that needs low-quality nourishment. I additionally experienced

difficulty deciding my particular craving lines. Following a half year of week after week sessions, I don't think it is nonsensical to expect that I would completely comprehend and equipped for executing the natural eating rules without an idea.

2. Participation in this gathering didn't present to me any closer to find the reasons why I was an urgent and gorge eater. I had no answers. I accepted that I was eating for a type of uncertain horrendous mishap or relationship. Without any solutions for my conduct, I effectively sneaked out of the natural eating mentality soon after leaving the gathering.

In psychological conduct treatment, I found that my gorging and voraciously consuming food practices are responses to eating fewer carbs rules, or what I see as eating less junk food rule.

Things being what they are; the main motivation behind why intuitive eating didn't work for me is that there are seven guidelines to pursue and renegade against:

- Eat just when you are ravenous? I'll eat at whatever point I need.

- Eat what your body needs? Disregard eating healthy, I'll eat low-quality nourishment.

- Eat without interruptions? I'll eat before the TV on the off chance that I need to.

- Eat until fulfilled? I'll eat a couple of significant pieces more than fulfilled without cause.

- Eat with pleasure? I'm too bustling sitting in front of the TV and eating down various servings of cream chocolate to appreciate it.

- Eat plunking down in a quiet domain? All things considered, I'll eat my McChicken combo in the vehicle if I need to.

- Eat-in full perspective on others? I'll eat well nourishment before others, yet in the event that I need to pig out, I'll conceal my case of Oreos in my work area.

Again, it's winner-take-all, diet mindset. I needed to pursue totally, or there was no reason for attempting by any stretch of the imagination. Presently I realize that I gorge and gorge to defy years/many years of eating less junk food. Therefore, I've needed to modify my thoughts on weight reduction.

I needed to think of my own arrangement of rules. Also, thinking back on it, amusing enough, I figure I may have really turned into an instinctive eater coincidentally. I eat when I'm hungry (generally). I currently perceive the more unpretentious indications of craving (powerlessness to center, considerations float to nourishment), and I am set up with a solid bite.

I eat until I'm fulfilled. Some way or another, through the CBT procedure, I don't appear to require nourishment as much any longer rationally. This is an aftereffect of disclosing to myself that I can have it if I truly need it. I eat what my body needs (for the most part). I'm eating bunches of vegetables and natural products. I anticipate eating more advantageous supper choices.

Since I've persuaded myself that I can eat whatever I need, it removed the enchantment from "terrible" fat and sugary nourishments. If I have "awful" nourishment at times, I don't stress over it and proceed. Concerning other guidelines (eat with delight, eat plunking down in a quiet domain, eat without interruption, and eat in full perspective on others), I would state that I currently accomplish those things normally.

I make the most of my nourishment all the more now since I'm no longer in a free for all to get to the following piece. I will eat a baggie of goldfish in the vehicle; however, the requirement for voraciously consuming food has diminished drastically, so I never again want to gorge in the vehicle. Now that I have little ones, we only occasionally have the TV on at mealtimes, yet I additionally don't stress over it if I have a bite while viewing the Bachelorette. It's unwinding; I make the most of my tidbit; however, it's not thoughtless either. Furthermore, in conclusion, since the requirement for gorging has diminished, I don't want to eat in mystery.

In this way, there you have it. I didn't completely see every one of the standards, and the gathering treatment didn't assist me in finding any solutions regarding why I gorged and gorged on nourishment. It is a challenge that ought not to be fooled with. The dietary propensities you grow now will be difficult to change in the coming years when your body stops creating, and your lifestyle may end up being progressively stationary. Making sense of how to choose sensible choices from a bewildering bunch of decisions isn't straightforward, despite that the prizes are incredible. Eating nutritious and refreshing nourishment keeping up your proper body weight, will add to an unrivaled display in the investigation hall, in the gym Centre, and on the rock floor. You will feel and put your best self forward.

Despite the fact that intuitive eating explicitly dismisses weight reduction, it may, in reality, help an individual shed a couple of pounds. For example, a few specialists have demonstrated that natural eating is related to lower BMI. "This is significant for wellbeing specialists who are worried that giving individuals a chance to eat whatever nourishment they want (genuine authorization to eat) would prompt weight gain," Evelyn Tribole recognizes.

In any case, she alerts that advancing intuitive eating as a technique for weight reduction can undermine and meddle with the procedure—and even reverse discharge on the individuals who attempt it. "if that a wellbeing expert or mentor is offering you intuitive eating with the end goal of weight reduction—flee quickly, "conversely, a terrible eating routine can prompt treacherous medical issues that can meddle with accomplishment in scholarly and social execution and may, in the end, mean facing a genuine long-haul sickness, for example, coronary illness or diabetes. Knowing how much and what to eat is significant learning.

Made in the USA
Coppell, TX
26 December 2019

13780324R00120